MW00991702

DENTAL ANATOMY

COLORING BOOK

DENTAL ANATOMY

COLORING BOOK

Edited by

Margaret J. Fehrenbach, RDH, MS
Educational Consultant and Private Practice
Seattle, Washington

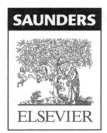

SAUNDERS

ELSEVIER

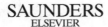

11830 Westline Industrial Drive
St. Louis, Missouri 63146

DENTAL ANATOMY COLORING BOOK ISBN 978-1-4160-4789-6

Copyright © 2008 by Saunders, an imprint of Elsevier Inc.

All rights reserved. No part of this publication may be reproduced or transmitted in any form or by any means, electronic or mechanical, including photocopying, recording, or any information storage and retrieval system, without permission in writing from the publisher.
Permissions may be sought directly from Elsevier's Health Sciences Rights Department in Philadelphia, PA, USA: phone: (+1) 215 239 3804, fax: (+1) 215 239 3805, e-mail: healthpermissions@elsevier.com. You may also complete your request on-line via the Elsevier homepage (http://www.elsevier.com), by selecting 'Customer Support' and then 'Obtaining Permissions'.

Notice

Neither the Publisher nor the Editor assumes any responsibility for any loss or injury and/or damage to persons or property arising out of or related to any use of the material contained in this book. It is the responsibility of the treating practitioner, relying on independent expertise and knowledge of the patient, to determine the best treatment and method of application for the patient.

The Publisher

Library of Congress Control Number 2007929922

ISBN: 978-1-4160-4789-6

Publisher: Linda Duncan
Senior Editor: John Dolan
Developmental Editor: Courtney Sprehe
Publishing Services Manager: Patricia Tannian
Senior Designer: Andrea Lutes

Working together to grow
libraries in developing countries

www.elsevier.com | www.bookaid.org | www.sabre.org

ELSEVIER   BOOK AID International   Sabre Foundation

Printed in the United States of America

Last digit is the print number: 9 8 7 6 5

PREFACE

A thorough understanding of head and neck anatomy is vital for today's dental professional, and *Dental Anatomy Coloring Book* is an ideal companion for anyone studying dental anatomy and physiology. This book has been designed not only to help you identify different structures, but also to test your anatomical knowledge of the entire head and neck. Every dental professional needs to know the facial landmarks, veins, arteries, nerves, bones, and muscles of the head and neck region, and this *all-new* resource enhances learning and memory retention in an easy-to-use, FUN format.

Dental Anatomy Coloring Book delivers complete anatomical coverage of the head and neck, beginning with an overview of the body and then moving to specific areas of the head and neck, including the dentition, skeletal system, muscles, and much more. This book will help you to visually understand the different parts of the head and neck and the impact of these parts on one another. One of the most effective ways for students to learn about the intricacies of the human body is by coloring detailed illustrations of various body parts. Use and review this book before an exam, before a class, or even before seeing your next patient.

Coloring is being used in formal therapeutic settings to develop eye-hand coordination, reduce stress, and help heal victims of trauma. Regardless of your needs, much can be gained by spending some time coloring. Choosing your colors and gently, repetitively moving your hand as you bring color to paper help to quiet your mind—bringing your usual rapid-fire thoughts down to a much slower pace. So take a break from your studies and find your creative center.

HOW TO USE THE BOOK

Each page contains a brief statement describing the body part featured and its orientation view, followed by a crisp, easy-to-color illustration. Numbered leader lines clearly identify the structures to be colored and correspond to a numbered list appearing below the illustration. You can create your own "color code" by using the same color to fill in the boxed number appearing on the illustration, the anatomical structure, and the corresponding numbered box on the list below the illustration. An example of a completed illustration can be found on the inside front cover.

ACKNOWLEDGMENTS

We would like to acknowledge the use of the following books as a basis for the creation of this text, as well as the figures drawn by Pat Thomas, CMI, Medical Illustrator, that appeared in some of these books.

- Applegate E: The Anatomy and Physiology Learning System, ed 3, Philadelphia, Saunders, 2006.
- Bath-Balogh M, Fehrenbach MJ: Illustrated Dental Embryology, Histology, and Anatomy, ed 2, St. Louis, Saunders, 2006.
- Fehrenbach MJ, Herring SW: Illustrated Anatomy of the Head and Neck, ed 3, St. Louis, Saunders, 2007.
- Norton NS: Netter's Head and Neck Anatomy for Dentistry, Philadelphia, Saunders, 2007.

CONTENTS

Copyright © 2008 by Saunders, an imprint of Elsevier Inc.

Copyright © 2008 by Saunders, an imprint of Elsevier Inc.

Contents

Copyright © 2008 by Saunders, an imprint of Elsevier Inc.

FIGURE 1-1 | Body sections and planes (anatomical position)

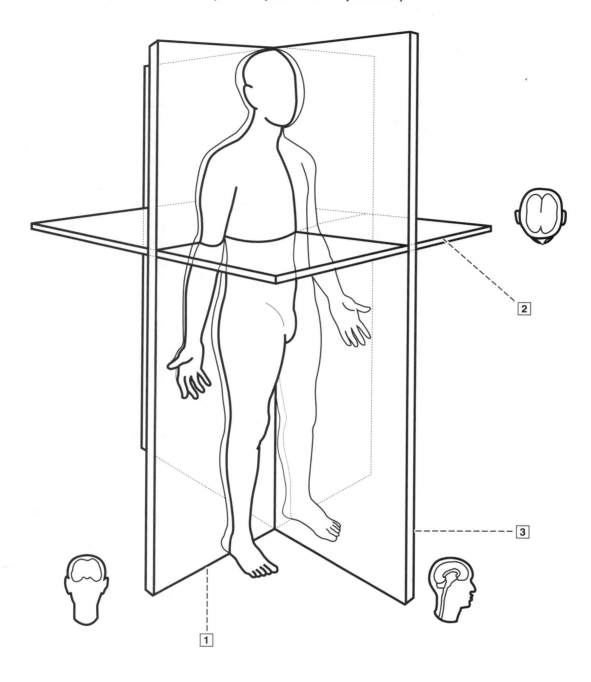

1	Frontal (coronal) section Frontal plane
2	Transverse section Horizontal plane
3	Midsagittal section Median plane

Copyright © 2008 by Saunders, an imprint of Elsevier Inc.

NOTES

Copyright © 2008 by Saunders, an imprint of Elsevier Inc.

FIGURE 1-2 | Major body cavities (midsagittal section)

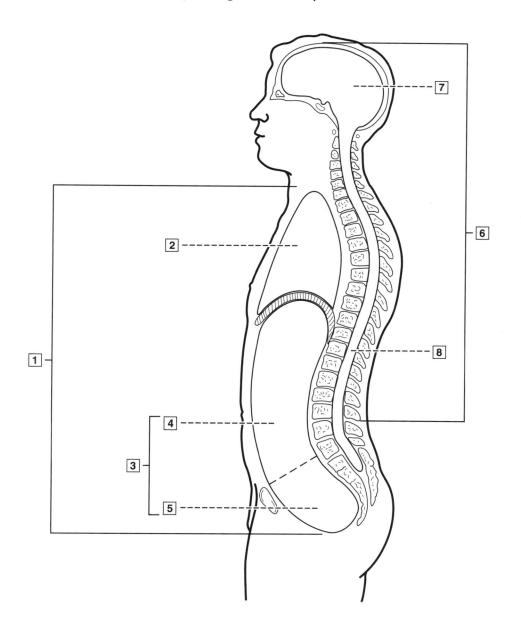

1	Ventral cavity	**5**	Pelvic cavity
2	Thoracic cavity	**6**	Dorsal cavity
3	Abdominopelvic cavity	**7**	Cranial cavity
4	Abdominal cavity	**8**	Spinal cavity

Copyright © 2008 by Saunders, an imprint of Elsevier Inc.

NOTES

Copyright © 2008 by Saunders, an imprint of Elsevier Inc.

FIGURE 1-3 | Major bones (anterior and posterior views)

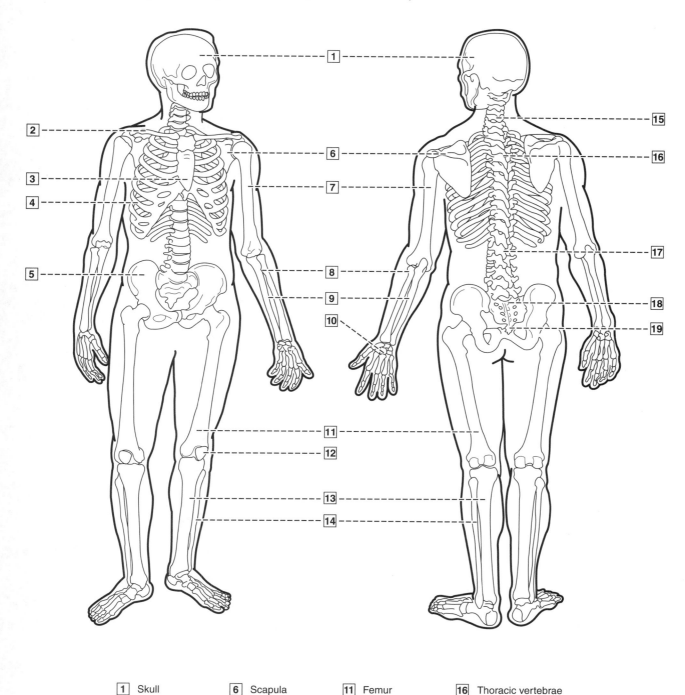

1 Skull	**6** Scapula	**11** Femur	**16** Thoracic vertebrae
2 Clavicle	**7** Humerus	**12** Patella	**17** Lumbar vertebrae
3 Sternum	**8** Radius	**13** Tibia	**18** Sacrum
4 Ribs	**9** Ulna	**14** Fibula	**19** Coccyx
5 Os coxae	**10** Carpals	**15** Verterbal column/ Cervical vertebrae	

Copyright © 2008 by Saunders, an imprint of Elsevier Inc.

NOTES

Copyright © 2008 by Saunders, an imprint of Elsevier Inc.

FIGURE 1-4 | Bone (transverse and cutaway views)

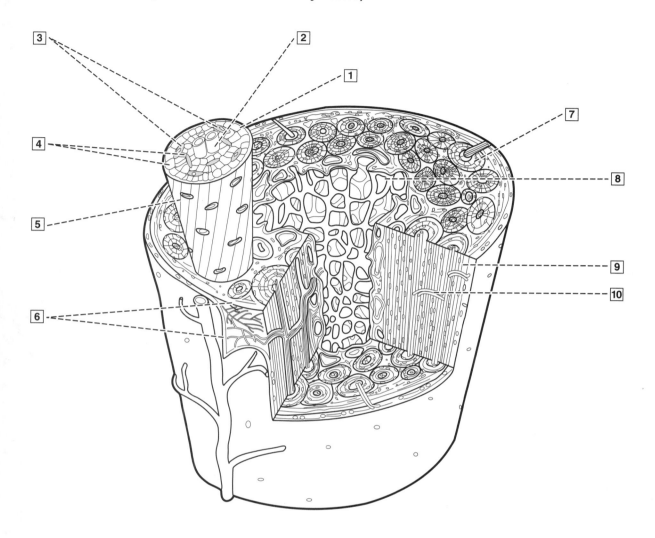

1. Lamellae
2. Haversian canal
3. Lacunae containing osteocytes
4. Canaliculi
5. Osteon
6. Periosteum
7. Osteon of compact bone
8. Trabeculae of spongy bone
9. Haversian canal
10. Volkmann's canal

Copyright © 2008 by Saunders, an imprint of Elsevier Inc.

NOTES

Copyright © 2008 by Saunders, an imprint of Elsevier Inc.

FIGURE 1-5 | Muscle tissue (transverse sections)

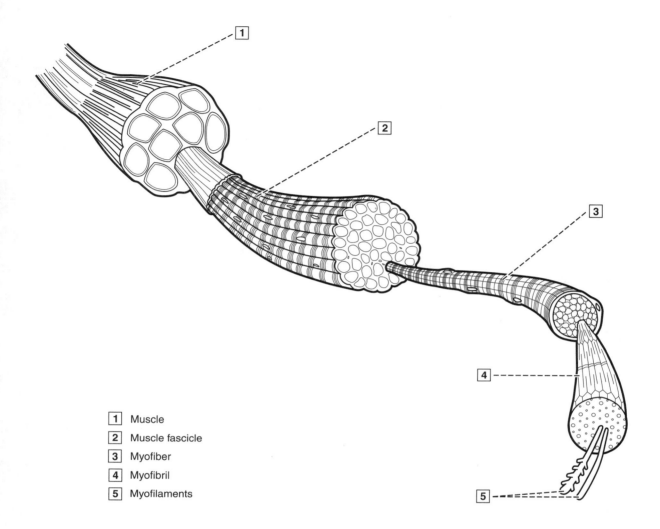

1 Muscle
2 Muscle fascicle
3 Myofiber
4 Myofibril
5 Myofilaments

Copyright © 2008 by Saunders, an imprint of Elsevier Inc.

NOTES

Copyright © 2008 by Saunders, an imprint of Elsevier Inc.

FIGURE 1-6 | Major body muscles (anterior view)

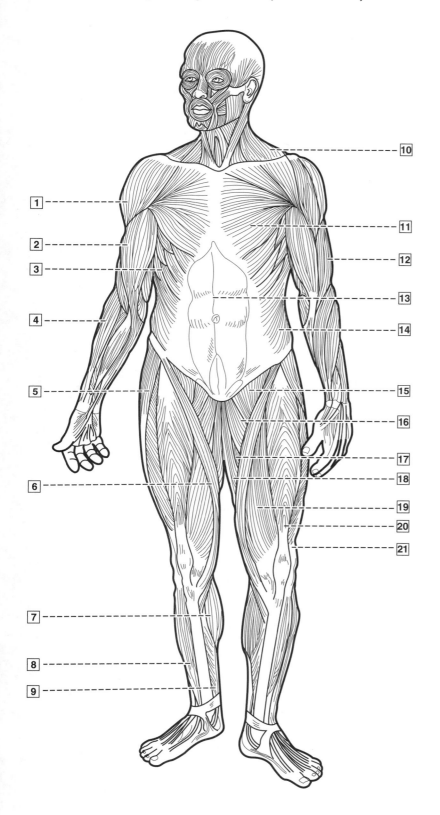

1	Deltoid
2	Biceps brachii
3	Serratus anterior
4	Brachioradialis
5	Tensor fasciae latae
6	Sartorius
7	Gastrocnemius
8	Tibialis anterior
9	Soleus
10	Trapezius
11	Pectoralis major
12	Brachialis
13	Linea alba
14	External abdominal oblique
15	Iliopsoas
16	Adductor longus
17	Adductor magnus
18	Gracilis
19	Vastus medialis
20	Rectus femoris
21	Vastus lateralis

Copyright © 2008 by Saunders, an imprint of Elsevier Inc.

NOTES

Copyright © 2008 by Saunders, an imprint of Elsevier Inc.

FIGURE 1-7 | Major body muscles (posterior view)

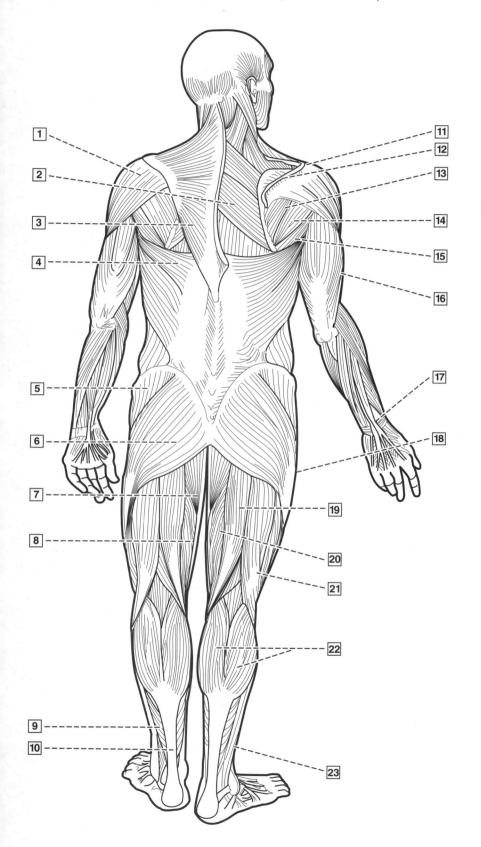

1	Deltoid
2	Rhomboideus major
3	Trapezius
4	Latissimus dorsi
5	Gluteus medius
6	Gluteus maximus
7	Adductor magnus
8	Gracilis
9	Soleus
10	Calcaneal tendon
11	Cut edge of trapezius
12	Supraspinatus
13	Infraspinatus
14	Teres minor
15	Teres major
16	Triceps brachii
17	Extensor digitorum
18	Tensor fasciae latae
19	Semitendinosus
20	Semimembranosus
21	Biceps femoris
22	Gastrocnemius
23	Peroneus longus

Copyright © 2008 by Saunders, an imprint of Elsevier Inc.

NOTES

Copyright © 2008 by Saunders, an imprint of Elsevier Inc.

FIGURE 1-8 | Blood vessels (transverse sections and cutaway view)

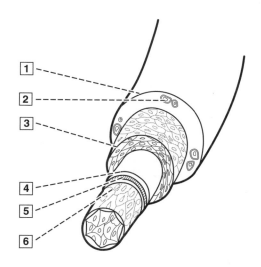

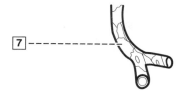

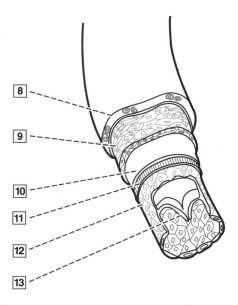

ARTERY

Tunica externa (adventitia)

1 Connective tissue
2 Vasa vasorum

Tunica media

3 Smooth muscle

Tunica intima

4 Elastic fibers
5 Basement membrane
6 Endothelium

CAPILLARY

7 Endothelium

VEIN

Tunica externa

8 Connective tissue

Tunica media

9 Smooth muscle

Tunica intima

10 Elastic fibers
11 Basement membrane
12 Endothelium
13 Venous valve

Copyright © 2008 by Saunders, an imprint of Elsevier Inc.

NOTES

Copyright © 2008 by Saunders, an imprint of Elsevier Inc.

FIGURE 1-9 | Major blood vessels and heart (frontal view)

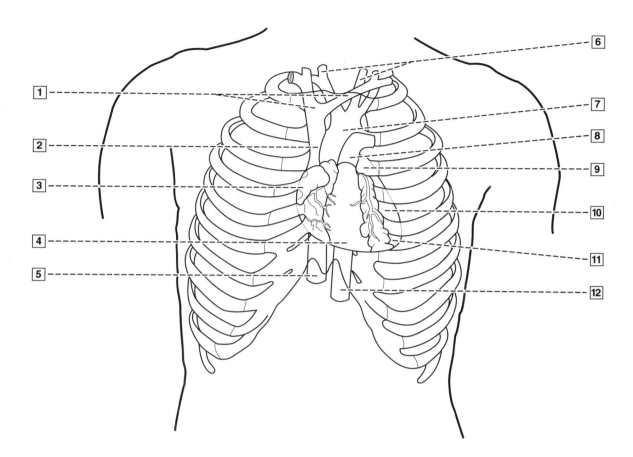

1	Brachiocephalic veins	7	Aorta (arch)
2	Superior vena cava	8	Pulmonary trunk
3	Right atrium	9	Left atrial appendage
4	Right ventricle	10	Left ventricle
5	Inferior vena cava	11	Apex
6	Common carotid arteries	12	Aorta (thoracic)

Copyright © 2008 by Saunders, an imprint of Elsevier Inc.

NOTES

Copyright © 2008 by Saunders, an imprint of Elsevier Inc.

FIGURE 1-10 | Heart (internal view)

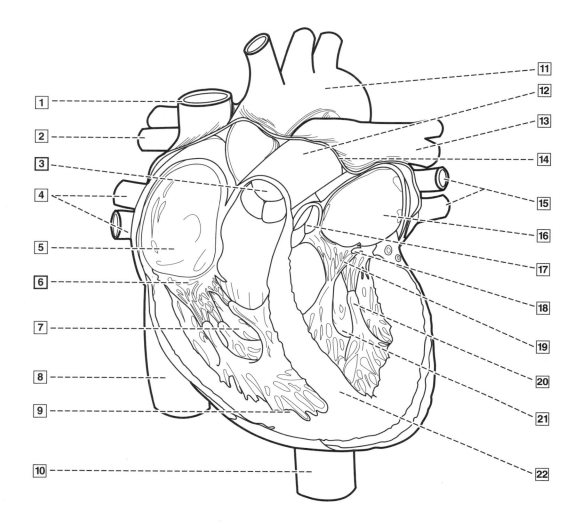

1	Superior vena cava	8	Inferior vena cava	15	Pulmonary veins	
2	Pulmonary arteries	9	Trabeculae carneae	16	Left atrium	
3	**Pulmonic valve**	10	Aorta (thoracic)	17	**Aortic valve**	
4	Pulmonary veins	11	Aorta (arch)	18	**Mitral (AV) valve**	
5	Right atrium	12	Pulmonary trunk	19	Chordae tendineae	
6	**Tricuspid (AV) valve**	13	Pulmonary artery	20	Papillary muscle	
7	Right ventricle	14	Cut edge of pericardium	21	Left ventricle	
				22	Interventricular septum	

Copyright © 2008 by Saunders, an imprint of Elsevier Inc.

NOTES

Copyright © 2008 by Saunders, an imprint of Elsevier Inc.

FIGURE 1-11 | Major systemic arteries (frontal view)

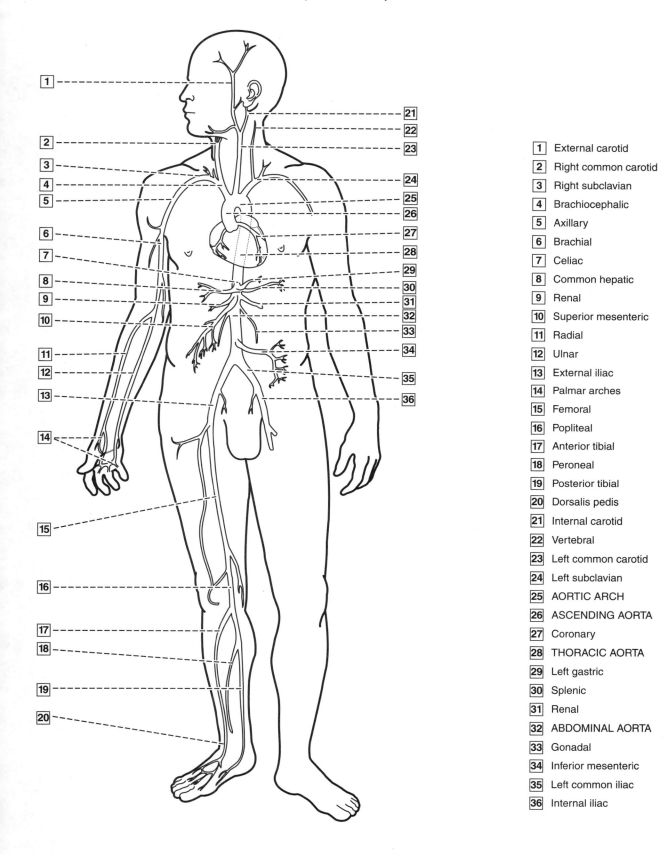

1	External carotid
2	Right common carotid
3	Right subclavian
4	Brachiocephalic
5	Axillary
6	Brachial
7	Celiac
8	Common hepatic
9	Renal
10	Superior mesenteric
11	Radial
12	Ulnar
13	External iliac
14	Palmar arches
15	Femoral
16	Popliteal
17	Anterior tibial
18	Peroneal
19	Posterior tibial
20	Dorsalis pedis
21	Internal carotid
22	Vertebral
23	Left common carotid
24	Left subclavian
25	AORTIC ARCH
26	ASCENDING AORTA
27	Coronary
28	THORACIC AORTA
29	Left gastric
30	Splenic
31	Renal
32	ABDOMINAL AORTA
33	Gonadal
34	Inferior mesenteric
35	Left common iliac
36	Internal iliac

Copyright © 2008 by Saunders, an imprint of Elsevier Inc.

NOTES

Copyright © 2008 by Saunders, an imprint of Elsevier Inc.

FIGURE 1-12 | Major systemic veins (frontal view)

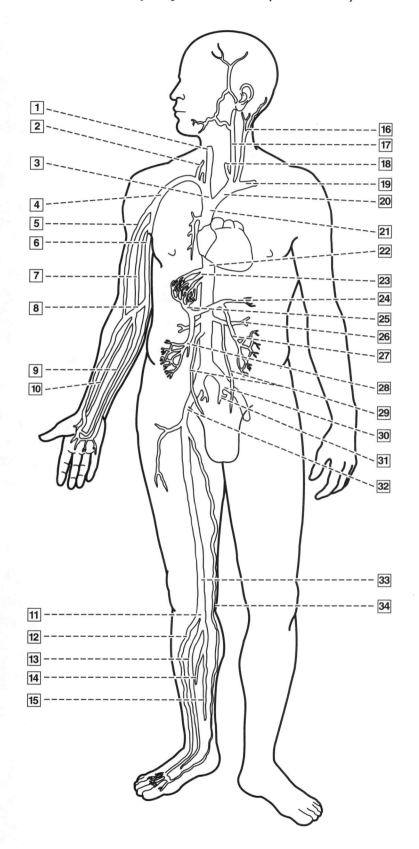

1	Right internal jugular
2	Right external jugular
3	Right brachiocephalic
4	Axillary
5	Cephalic
6	Basilic
7	Brachial
8	Median cubital
9	Ulnar
10	Radial
11	Popliteal
12	Small saphenous
13	Anterior tibial
14	Peroneal
15	Posterior tibial
16	Left external jugular
17	Left internal jugular
18	Vertebral
19	Subclavian
20	Left brachiocephalic
21	Superior vena cava
22	Inferior vena cava
23	Hepatic
24	Splenic
25	Hepatic portal
26	Renal
27	Inferior mesenteric
28	Superior mesenteric
29	Gonadal
30	Common iliac
31	Internal iliac
32	External iliac
33	Femoral
34	Great saphenous

Copyright © 2008 by Saunders, an imprint of Elsevier Inc.

NOTES

Copyright © 2008 by Saunders, an imprint of Elsevier Inc.

FIGURE 1-13 | Upper and lower respiratory tract (midsagittal section and frontal and cutaway views)

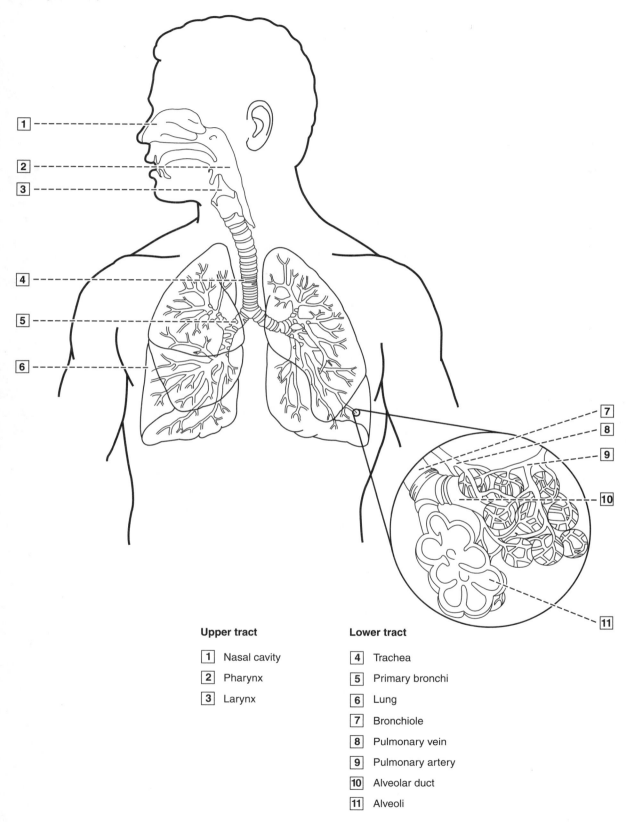

Upper tract

1. Nasal cavity
2. Pharynx
3. Larynx

Lower tract

4. Trachea
5. Primary bronchi
6. Lung
7. Bronchiole
8. Pulmonary vein
9. Pulmonary artery
10. Alveolar duct
11. Alveoli

Copyright © 2008 by Saunders, an imprint of Elsevier Inc.

NOTES

Copyright © 2008 by Saunders, an imprint of Elsevier Inc.

FIGURE 1-14 | Endocrine glands (midsagittal section and frontal, posterior, and close-up views)

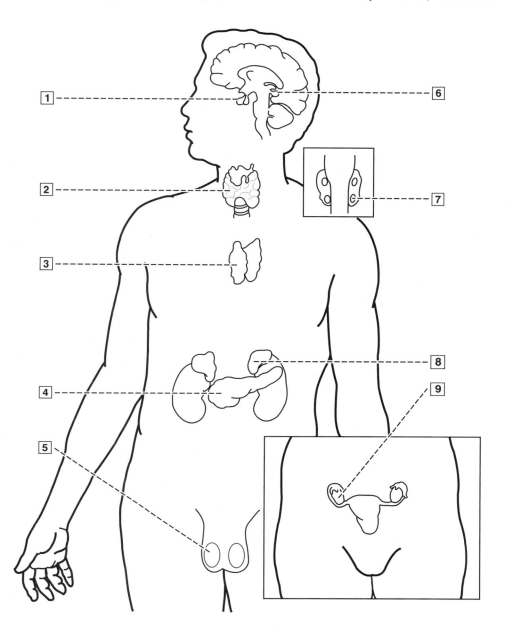

1	Pituitary gland	6	Pineal gland
2	Thyroid gland	7	Parathyroid gland (on posterior surface of thyroid gland)
3	Thymus		
4	Pancreas	8	Adrenal gland
5	Testis	9	Ovary

Copyright © 2008 by Saunders, an imprint of Elsevier Inc.

NOTES

Copyright © 2008 by Saunders, an imprint of Elsevier Inc.

FIGURE 1-15 | Digestive system (midsagittal section and frontal view)

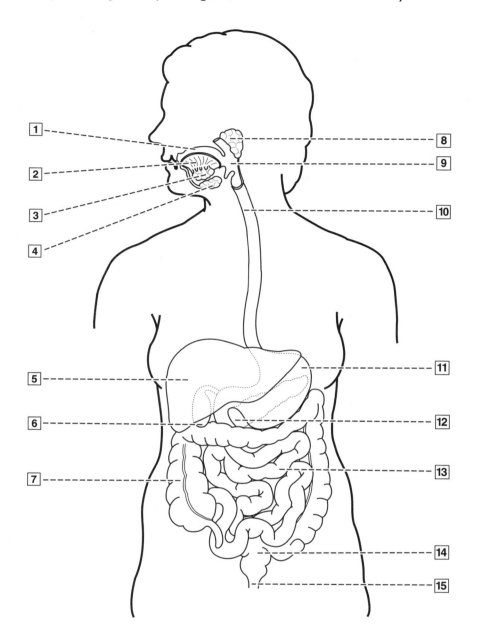

1	Mouth (oral cavity)	6	Gallbladder	11	Stomach
2	Tongue	7	Large intestine	12	Pancreas
3	Sublingual salivary gland	8	Parotid salivary gland	13	Small intestine
4	Submandibular salivary gland	9	Pharynx	14	Rectum
5	Liver	10	Esophagus	15	Anus

Copyright © 2008 by Saunders, an imprint of Elsevier Inc.

NOTES

Copyright © 2008 by Saunders, an imprint of Elsevier Inc.

FIGURE 1-16 | Urinary system (frontal view)

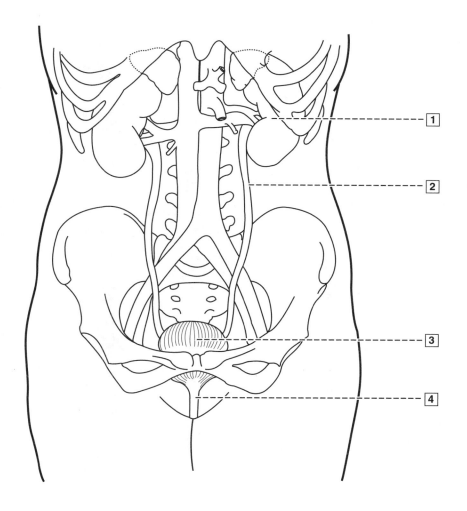

1	Kidney	**3**	Bladder
2	Ureter	**4**	Urethra

Copyright © 2008 by Saunders, an imprint of Elsevier Inc.

NOTES

Copyright © 2008 by Saunders, an imprint of Elsevier Inc.

FIGURE 1-17 | Major lymphatics (sagittal section)

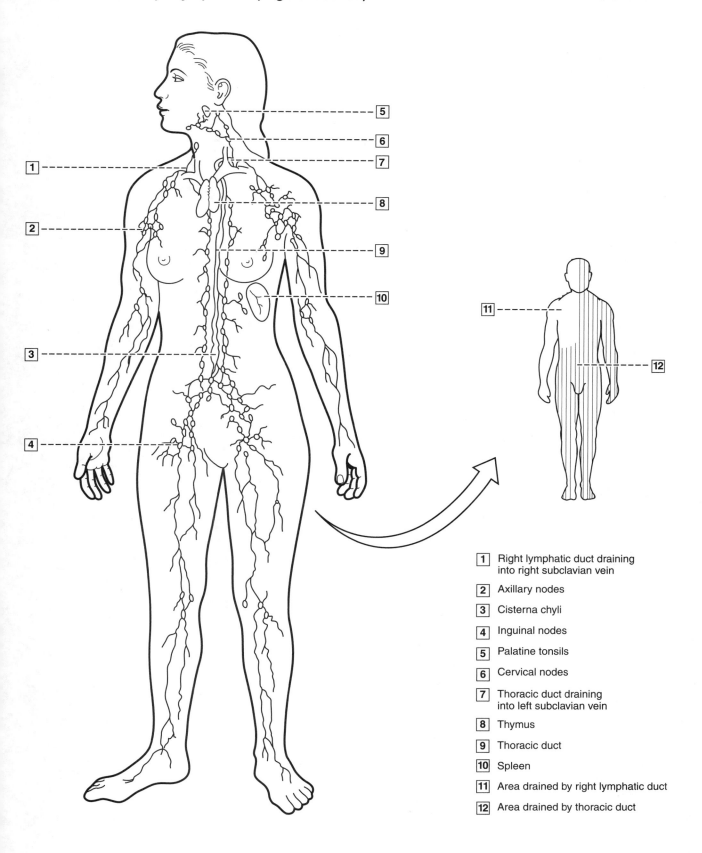

1	Right lymphatic duct draining into right subclavian vein
2	Axillary nodes
3	Cisterna chyli
4	Inguinal nodes
5	Palatine tonsils
6	Cervical nodes
7	Thoracic duct draining into left subclavian vein
8	Thymus
9	Thoracic duct
10	Spleen
11	Area drained by right lymphatic duct
12	Area drained by thoracic duct

Copyright © 2008 by Saunders, an imprint of Elsevier Inc.

NOTES

Copyright © 2008 by Saunders, an imprint of Elsevier Inc.

FIGURE 1-18 | Lymph node (sagittal section)

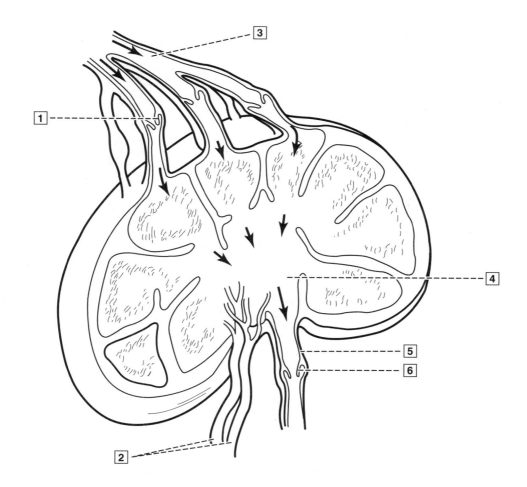

1	Valve	4	Hilus
2	Blood vessels	5	Efferent lymphatic vessels
3	Afferent lymphatic vessels	6	Valve

Copyright © 2008 by Saunders, an imprint of Elsevier Inc.

NOTES

Copyright © 2008 by Saunders, an imprint of Elsevier Inc.

FIGURE 1-19 | Central and peripheral nervous systems

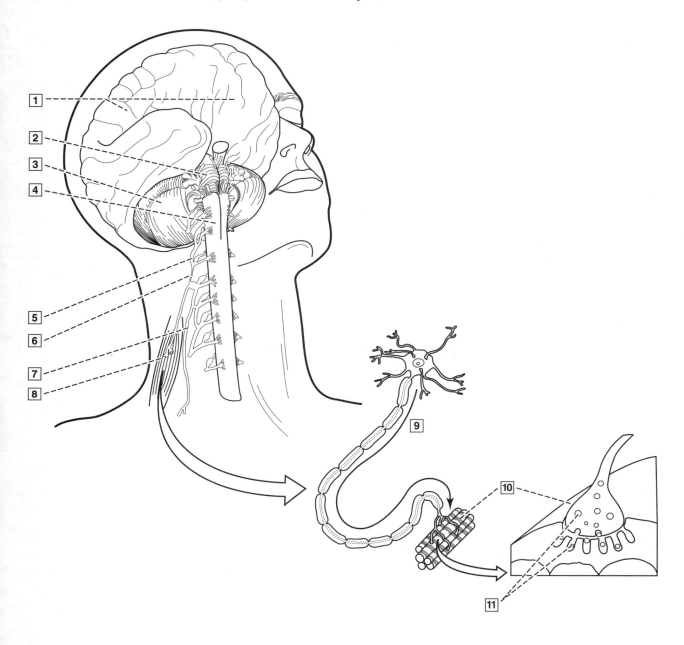

Central nervous system

1 Cerebrum

2 Brainstem

3 Cerebellum

4 Spinal cord

Peripheral nervous system

5 Nerve ganglion

6 Nerve

7 Afferent nerve from skin

8 Efferent nerve to muscle

Neuron

9 Action potential (impulse propagation)

10 Muscle fiber

Synapse

10 Muscle fiber

11 Neurotransmitter

Copyright © 2008 by Saunders, an imprint of Elsevier Inc.

NOTES

Copyright © 2008 by Saunders, an imprint of Elsevier Inc.

FIGURE 1-20 | Neuron

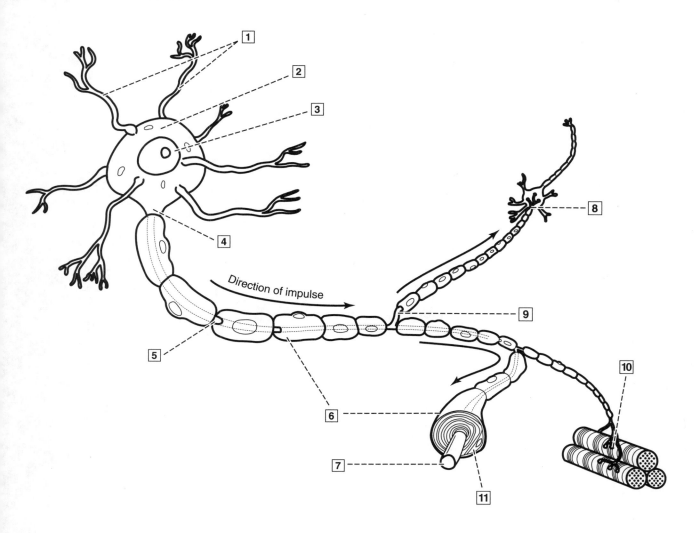

Direction of impulse

1 Dendrites	**7** Axon
2 Cell body	**8** Synapse with another neuron
3 Nucleus	**9** Collateral branch
4 Axon	**10** Synapse with myofibers
5 Node of Ranvier	**11** Nucleus of Schwann cell
6 Myelin sheath	

Copyright © 2008 by Saunders, an imprint of Elsevier Inc.

NOTES

Copyright © 2008 by Saunders, an imprint of Elsevier Inc.

FIGURE 2-1 | Head and neck sections and planes (anatomical position)

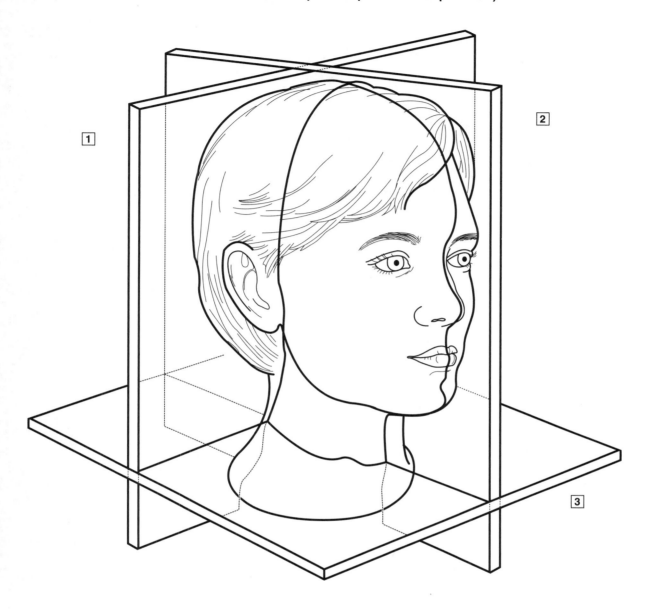

1 Frontal (coronal) section/Frontal plane

2 Midsagittal section/Median plane

3 Transverse section/Horizontal plane

Copyright © 2008 by Saunders, an imprint of Elsevier Inc.

NOTES

Copyright © 2008 by Saunders, an imprint of Elsevier Inc.

FIGURE 2-2 | Regions of the head (frontal view)

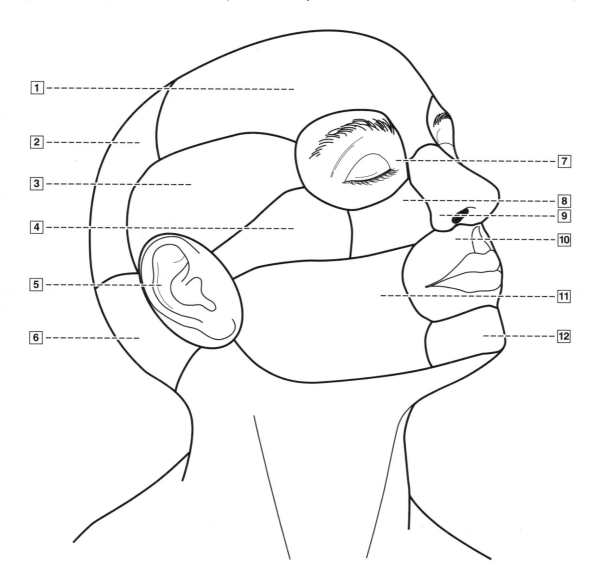

1	Frontal region		7	Orbital region
2	Parietal region		8	Infraorbital region
3	Temporal region		9	Nasal region
4	Zygomatic region		10	Oral region
5	Auricular region		11	Buccal region
6	Occipital region		12	Mental region

Copyright © 2008 by Saunders, an imprint of Elsevier Inc.

NOTES

Copyright © 2008 by Saunders, an imprint of Elsevier Inc.

FIGURE 2-3 | Frontal region: head (frontal view)

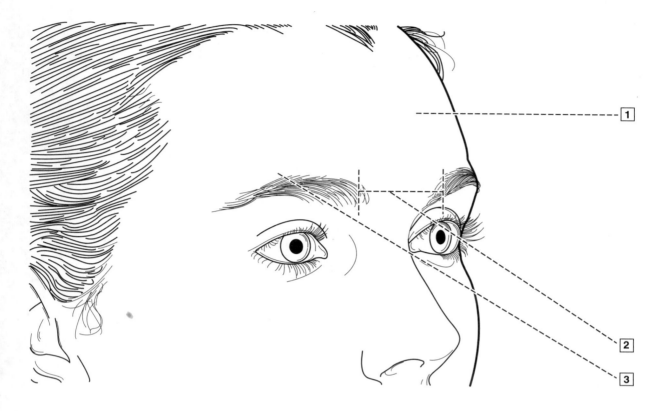

1 Frontal eminence

2 Glabella

3 Supraorbital ridge

Copyright © 2008 by Saunders, an imprint of Elsevier Inc.

NOTES

Copyright © 2008 by Saunders, an imprint of Elsevier Inc.

FIGURE 2-4 | Auricular region: external ear (lateral view)

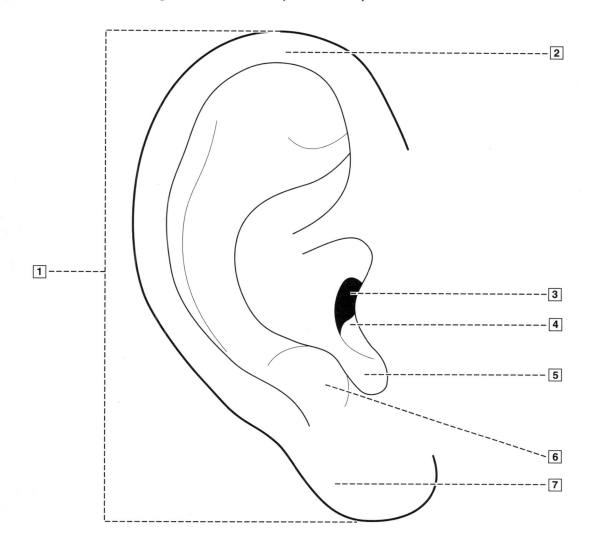

1	Auricle	5	Intertragic notch
2	Helix	6	Antitragus
3	External acoustic meatus	7	Lobule
4	Tragus		

Copyright © 2008 by Saunders, an imprint of Elsevier Inc.

NOTES

Copyright © 2008 by Saunders, an imprint of Elsevier Inc.

FIGURE 2-5 | Orbital region: surface anatomy (frontal and internal views)

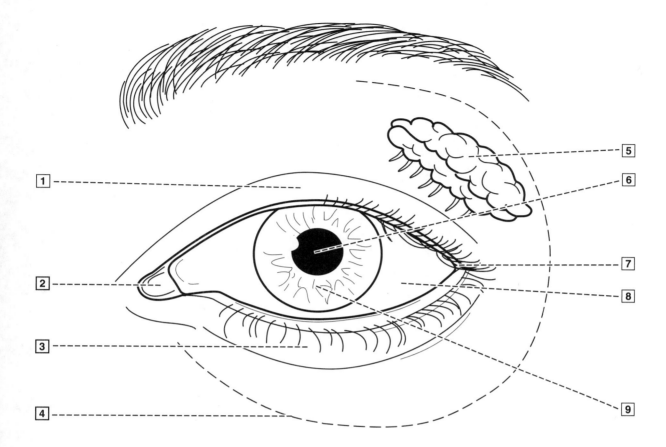

1 Upper eyelid		**7** Lateral canthus	
2 Medial canthus		**8** Sclera (covered by conjunctiva)	
3 Lower eyelid		**9** Iris	
4 Orbit (outlined)			
5 Lacrimal gland (deep)			
6 Pupil			

Copyright © 2008 by Saunders, an imprint of Elsevier Inc.

NOTES

Copyright © 2008 by Saunders, an imprint of Elsevier Inc.

FIGURE 2-6 | Orbital region: eye (sagittal section)

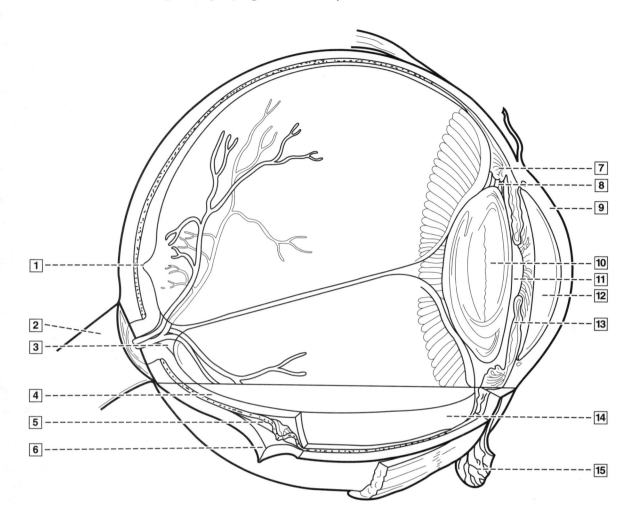

1 Fovea centralis	6 Sclera	11 Pupil
2 Optic nerve	7 Ciliary body	12 Anterior cavity filled with aqueous humor
3 Optic disk	8 Suspensory ligament	13 Iris
4 Retina	9 Cornea	14 Vitreous humor
5 Choroid	10 Lens	15 Conjunctiva

Copyright © 2008 by Saunders, an imprint of Elsevier Inc.

NOTES

Copyright © 2008 by Saunders, an imprint of Elsevier Inc.

FIGURE 2-7 ∣ Nasal region: surface anatomy (frontal view)

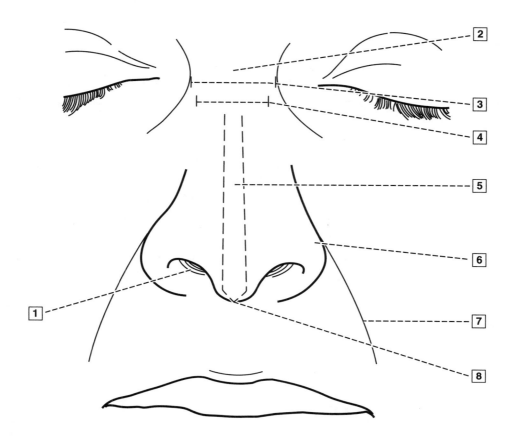

1	Naris	**5**	Nasal septum (outlined)
2	Nasion	**6**	Ala
3	Root of nose	**7**	Nasolabial sulcus
4	Bridge of nose	**8**	Apex

Copyright © 2008 by Saunders, an imprint of Elsevier Inc.

NOTES

Copyright © 2008 by Saunders, an imprint of Elsevier Inc.

FIGURE 2-8 | Nasal region: olfactory receptors (sagittal section and cutaway view)

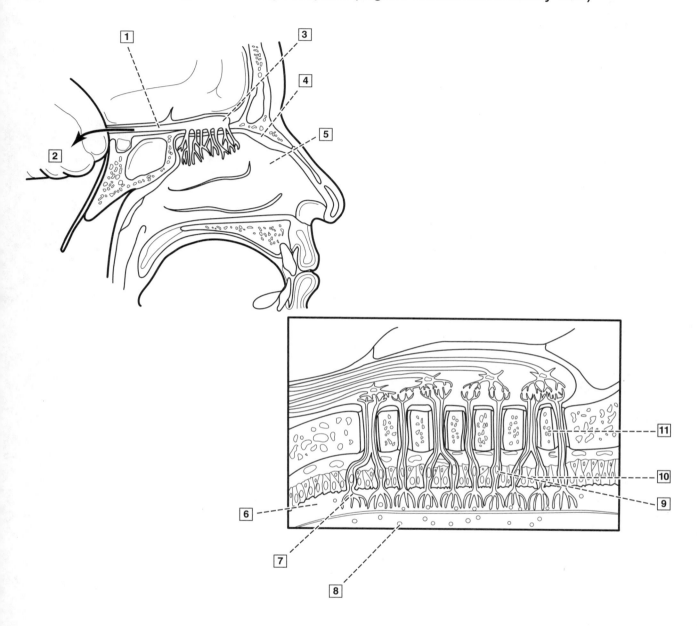

1	Olfactory tract	6	Mucous layer
2	Temporal lobe Olfactory cortex	7	Cilia of receptor cell
3	Olfactory bulb	8	Odor molecule
4	Olfactory epithelium	9	Cell body of olfactory neuron
5	Nasal cavity	10	Supporting cells
		11	Cribriform plate of ethmoid bone

Copyright © 2008 by Saunders, an imprint of Elsevier Inc.

NOTES

Copyright © 2008 by Saunders, an imprint of Elsevier Inc.

FIGURE 2-9 | Zygomatic, infraorbital, buccal, and mental regions: surface anatomy (frontal and internal views)

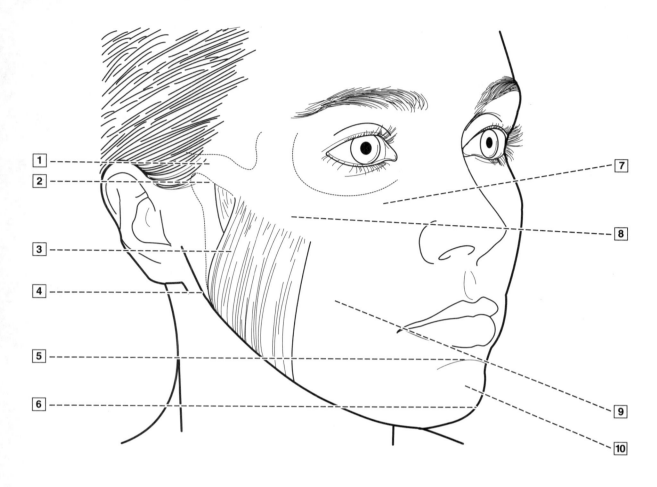

1	Zygomatic arch (deep)	6	Mental protuberance
2	Temporomandibular joint	7	Infraorbital region
3	Masseter muscle (deep)	8	Zygomatic region
4	Angle of mandible	9	Buccal region
5	Labiomental groove	10	Mental region

Copyright © 2008 by Saunders, an imprint of Elsevier Inc.

NOTES

Copyright © 2008 by Saunders, an imprint of Elsevier Inc.

FIGURE 2-10 | Oral region: lips (frontal view)

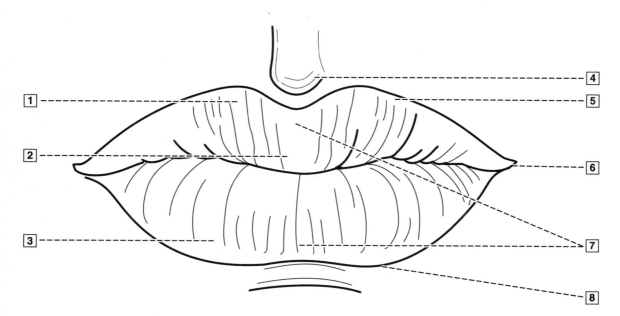

1 Upper lip		**6** Labial commissure	
2 Tubercle		**7** Vermilion zone	
3 Lower lip		**8** Vermilion border	
4 Philtrum			
5 Vermilion border			

Copyright © 2008 by Saunders, an imprint of Elsevier Inc.

NOTES

Copyright © 2008 by Saunders, an imprint of Elsevier Inc.

FIGURE 2-11 | Oral region: oral mucosa (lateral view)

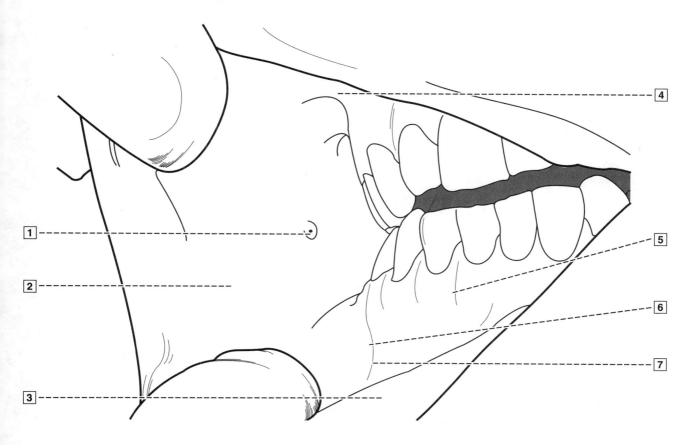

1	Parotid papilla	5	Alveolar mucosa
2	Buccal mucosa	6	Mucobuccal fold
3	Labial mucosa	7	Mandibular vestibule
4	Maxillary vestibule		

Copyright © 2008 by Saunders, an imprint of Elsevier Inc.

NOTES

Copyright © 2008 by Saunders, an imprint of Elsevier Inc.

FIGURE 2-12 | Oral region: oral cavity (frontal view)

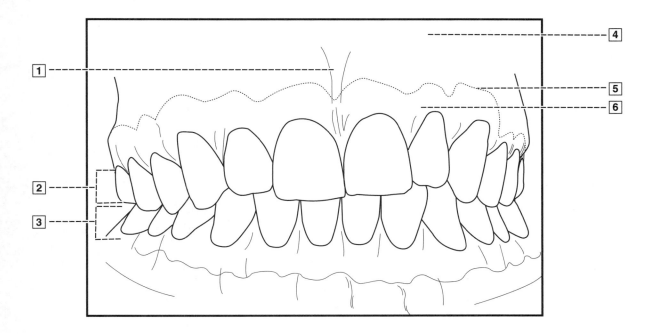

1	Labial frenum	4	Alveolar mucosa
2	Maxillary teeth	5	Mucogingival junction (outlined)
3	Mandibular teeth	6	Attached gingiva

Copyright © 2008 by Saunders, an imprint of Elsevier Inc.

NOTES

Copyright © 2008 by Saunders, an imprint of Elsevier Inc.

FIGURE 2-13 | Oral region: oral cavity—gingival tissues (frontal view)

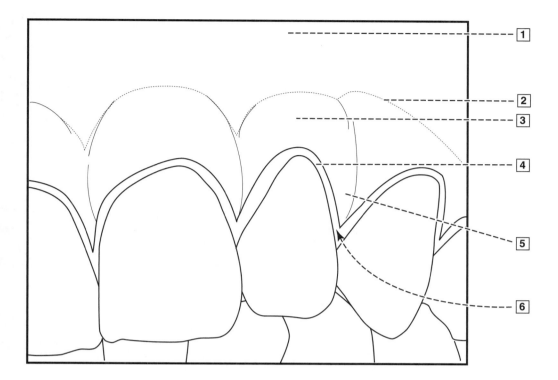

1 Alveolar mucosa	**4** Marginal gingiva
2 Mucogingival junction (outlined)	**5** Interdental gingiva
3 Attached gingiva	**6** Sulcus (inside)

Copyright © 2008 by Saunders, an imprint of Elsevier Inc.

NOTES

Copyright © 2008 by Saunders, an imprint of Elsevier Inc.

FIGURE 2-14 | Oral region: oral cavity—gingival tissues (oral mucosa)

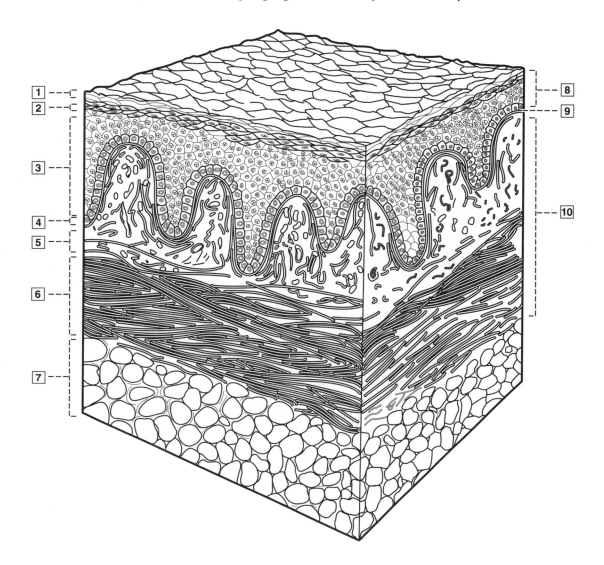

1	Keratin layer	**6**	Dense fibrous layer
2	Granular layer	**7**	Submucosa
3	Prickle layer	**8**	Oral epithelium
4	Basal layer	**9**	Basement membrane
5	Papillary layer	**10**	Lamina propria

Copyright © 2008 by Saunders, an imprint of Elsevier Inc.

NOTES

 Copyright © 2008 by Saunders, an imprint of Elsevier Inc.

FIGURE 2-15 | Oral region: oral cavity—gingival tissues (anatomy)

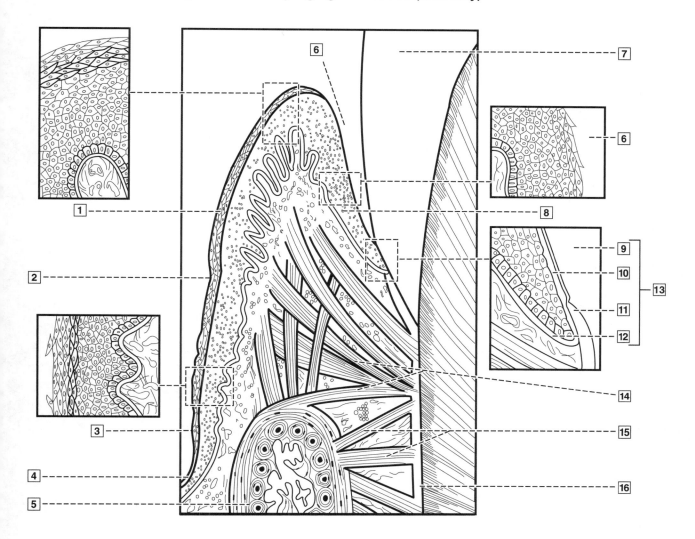

1	Marginal gingiva	9	Enamel
2	Free gingival groove	10	Internal basal lamina
3	Attached gingiva	11	Cementum
4	Alveolar mucosa	12	External basal lamina
5	Alveolar bone	13	Junctional epithelium
6	Gingival sulcus	14	Gingival fiber group
7	Tooth surface	15	Periodontal ligament
8	Sulcular epithelium	16	Cementum

Copyright © 2008 by Saunders, an imprint of Elsevier Inc.

NOTES

Copyright © 2008 by Saunders, an imprint of Elsevier Inc.

FIGURE 2-16 | Oral region: oral cavity—gingival tissues (junctional epithelium)

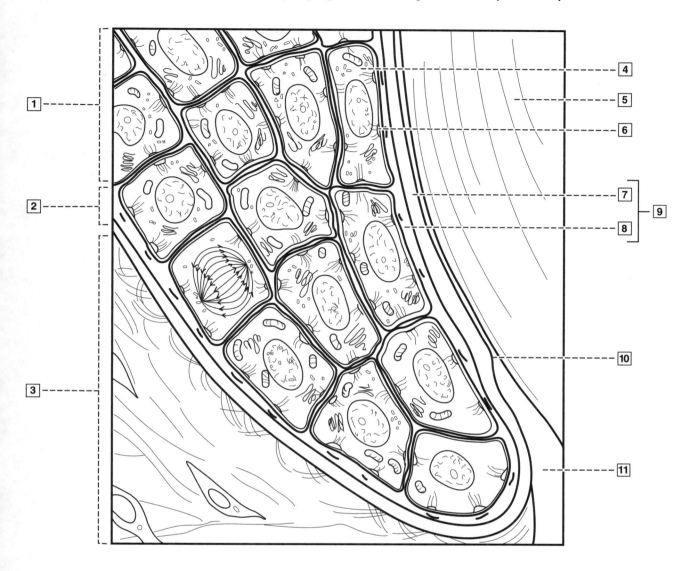

1 Basal layer	**7** Lamina densa	
2 External basal lamina	**8** Lamina lucida	
3 Lamina propria	**9** Internal basal lamina	
4 Junctional epithelial cell	**10** Cementoenamel junction	
5 Enamel	**11** Cementum	
6 Hemidesmosome		

Copyright © 2008 by Saunders, an imprint of Elsevier Inc.

NOTES

Copyright © 2008 by Saunders, an imprint of Elsevier Inc.

FIGURE 2-17 | Oral region: oral cavity—palate (inferior view)

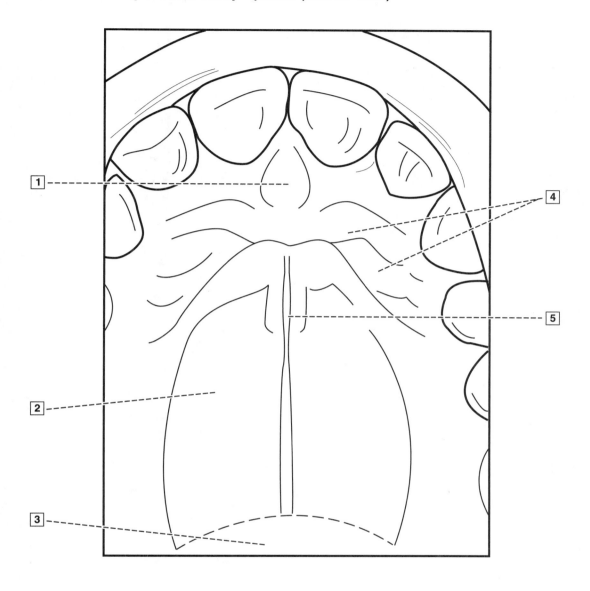

1 Incisive papilla
2 Hard palate
3 Soft palate
4 Palatine rugae
5 Median palatine raphe

Copyright © 2008 by Saunders, an imprint of Elsevier Inc.

NOTES

Copyright © 2008 by Saunders, an imprint of Elsevier Inc.

FIGURE 2-18 | Oral region: oral cavity—tongue (lateral view)

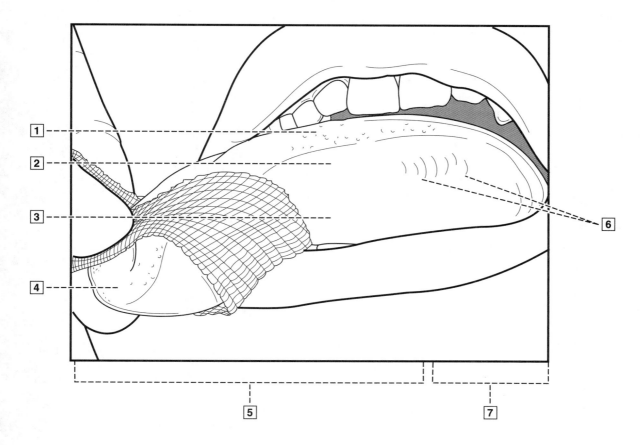

1	Dorsal surface	5	Body
2	Lateral surface	6	Foliate lingual papillae
3	Ventral surface	7	Base
4	Apex		

Copyright © 2008 by Saunders, an imprint of Elsevier Inc.

NOTES

Copyright © 2008 by Saunders, an imprint of Elsevier Inc.

FIGURE 2-19 | Oral region: oral cavity—tongue and taste buds (dorsal surface and close-up views)

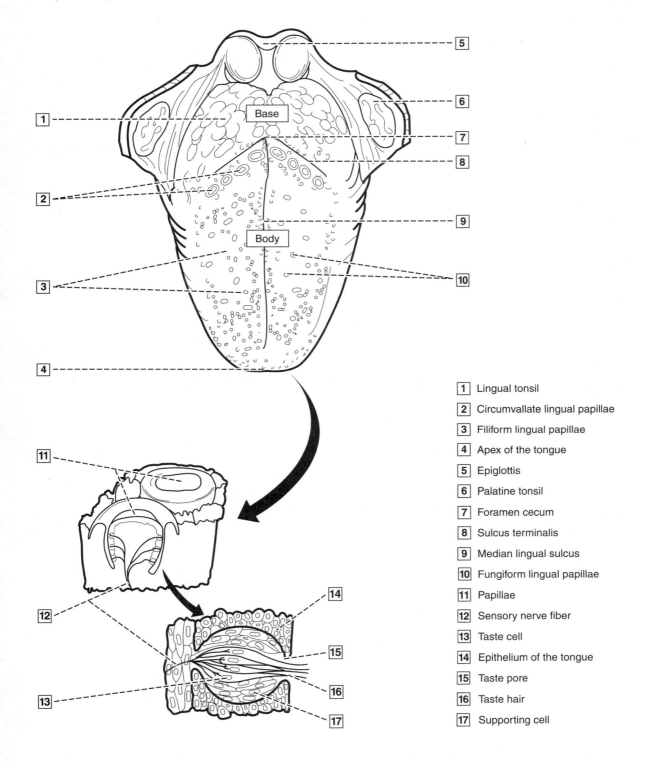

1 Lingual tonsil
2 Circumvallate lingual papillae
3 Filiform lingual papillae
4 Apex of the tongue
5 Epiglottis
6 Palatine tonsil
7 Foramen cecum
8 Sulcus terminalis
9 Median lingual sulcus
10 Fungiform lingual papillae
11 Papillae
12 Sensory nerve fiber
13 Taste cell
14 Epithelium of the tongue
15 Taste pore
16 Taste hair
17 Supporting cell

Copyright © 2008 by Saunders, an imprint of Elsevier Inc.

NOTES

Copyright © 2008 by Saunders, an imprint of Elsevier Inc.

FIGURE 2-20 | Oral region: oral cavity—tongue (ventral surface)

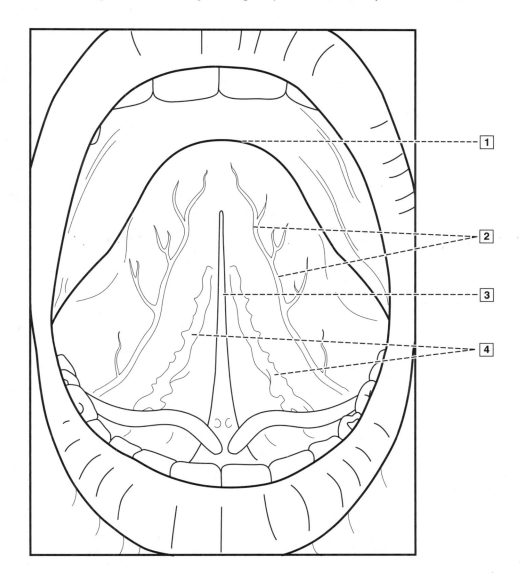

1 Apex
2 Deep lingual veins
3 Lingual frenum
4 Plicae fimbriatae

Copyright © 2008 by Saunders, an imprint of Elsevier Inc.

NOTES

Copyright © 2008 by Saunders, an imprint of Elsevier Inc.

FIGURE 2-21 | Oral region: oral cavity—floor of the mouth (superior view)

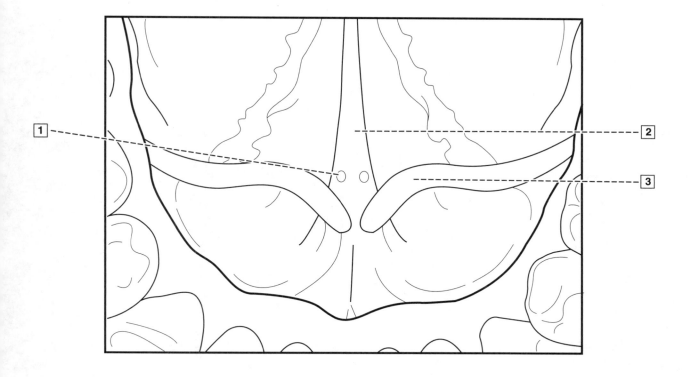

1 Sublingual caruncle
2 Lingual frenum
3 Sublingual fold

Copyright © 2008 by Saunders, an imprint of Elsevier Inc.

NOTES

Copyright © 2008 by Saunders, an imprint of Elsevier Inc.

FIGURE 2-22 | Pharynx and associated anatomy: surface anatomy (midsagittal section)

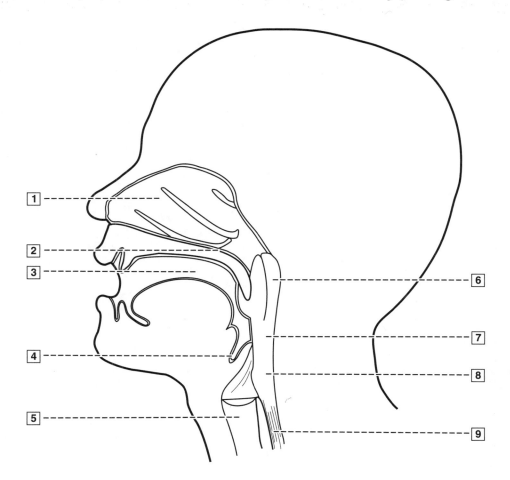

1	Nasal cavity	**6**	Nasopharynx
2	Soft palate	**7**	Oropharynx
3	Oral cavity	**8**	Laryngopharynx
4	Epiglottis	**9**	Esophagus
5	Larynx		

Copyright © 2008 by Saunders, an imprint of Elsevier Inc.

NOTES

Copyright © 2008 by Saunders, an imprint of Elsevier Inc.

FIGURE 2-23 | Oropharynx and associated anatomy: surface anatomy (frontal view)

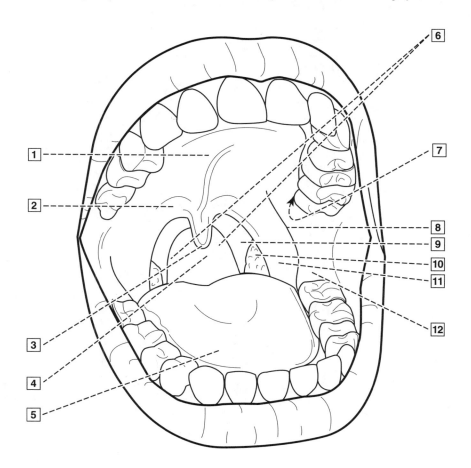

1 Hard palate	**7** Maxillary tuberosity
2 Soft palate	**8** Pterygomandibular fold
3 Uvula	**9** Posterior faucial pillar
4 Posterior wall of the pharynx	**10** Palatine tonsil
5 Dorsal surface of tongue	**11** Anterior faucial pillar
6 Fauces	**12** Retromandibular pad

Copyright © 2008 by Saunders, an imprint of Elsevier Inc.

NOTES

Copyright © 2008 by Saunders, an imprint of Elsevier Inc.

FIGURE 2-24 | Regions of the neck: surface anatomy (frontal view)

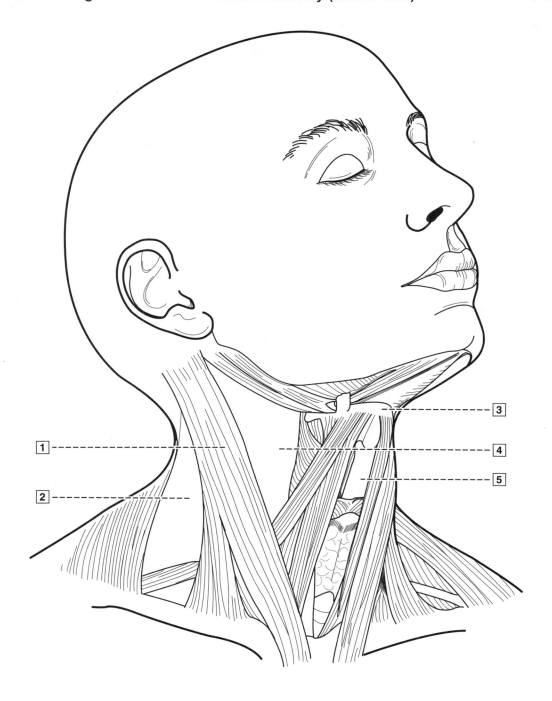

1 Sternocleidomastoid muscle 4 Anterior cervical triangle

2 Posterior cervical triangle 5 Thyroid cartilage

3 Hyoid bone

Copyright © 2008 by Saunders, an imprint of Elsevier Inc.

NOTES

Copyright © 2008 by Saunders, an imprint of Elsevier Inc.

FIGURE 2-25 | Regions of the neck: anterior cervical triangle (frontal view)

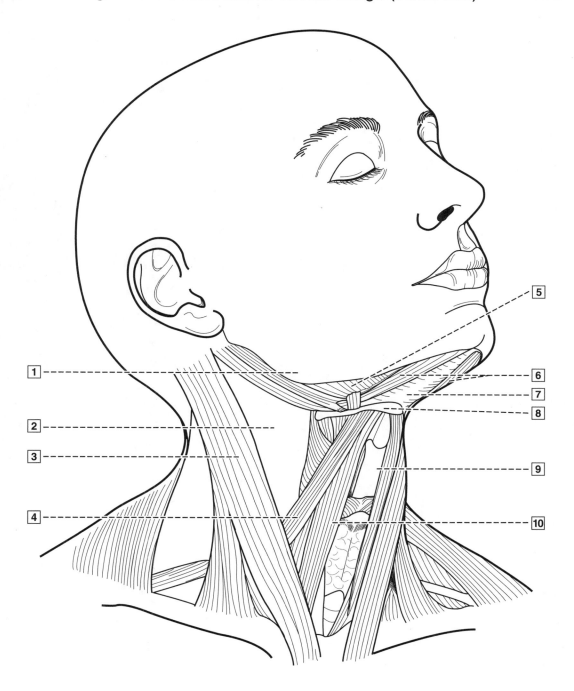

1	Mandible	6	Digastric muscles
2	Carotid triangle	7	Submental triangle
3	Sternocleidomastoid muscle	8	Hyoid bone
4	Omohyoid muscle	9	Thyroid cartilage
5	Submandibular triangle	10	Muscular triangle

Copyright © 2008 by Saunders, an imprint of Elsevier Inc.

NOTES

Copyright © 2008 by Saunders, an imprint of Elsevier Inc.

FIGURE 2-26 | Regions of the neck: posterior cervical triangle (frontal view)

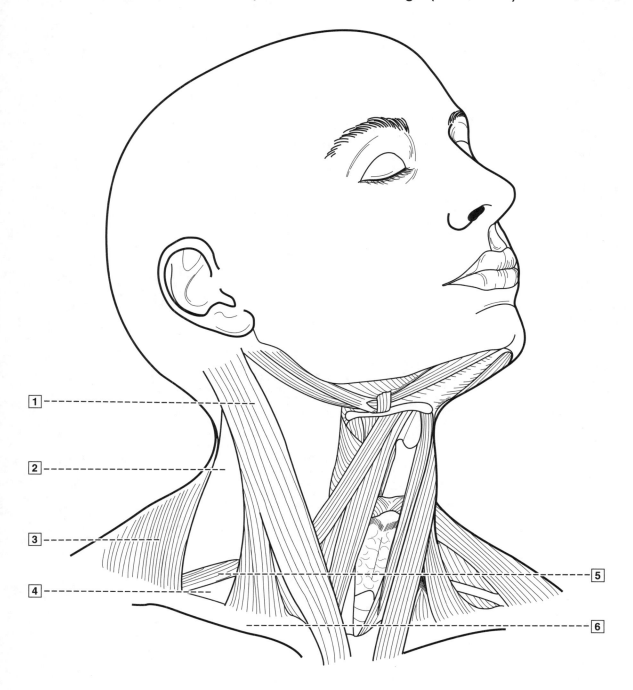

1 Sternocleidomastoid muscle   3 Trapezius muscle   5 Omohyoid muscle

2 Occipital triangle   4 Subclavian triangle   6 Clavicle

Copyright © 2008 by Saunders, an imprint of Elsevier Inc.

NOTES

Copyright © 2008 by Saunders, an imprint of Elsevier Inc.

FIGURE 3-1 │ The stages of tooth development (microscopic appearance)

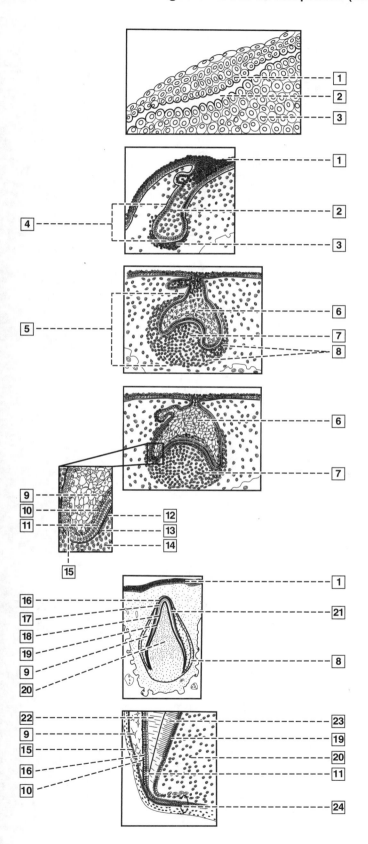

Initiation and bud stages

1 Oral epithelium

2 Dental lamina

3 Ectomesenchyme

4 Tooth bud

Cap stage

5 Tooth germ

6 Enamel organ

7 Dental papilla

8 Dental sac

Bell stage

9 Stellate reticulum

10 Stratum intermedium

11 Inner enamel epithelium

12 Basement membrane

13 Outer cells of the dental papilla

14 Central cells of the dental papilla

15 Outer enamel epithelium

Apposition stage

16 Ameloblasts

17 Enamel matrix

18 Dentin matrix

19 Odontoblasts

20 Pulp

21 Dentinoenamel junction

Maturation stage

22 Enamel

23 Dentin

24 Hertwig's epithelial root sheath

Copyright © 2008 by Saunders, an imprint of Elsevier Inc.

NOTES

Copyright © 2008 by Saunders, an imprint of Elsevier Inc.

FIGURE 3-2 | Primary and adult crown, root(s), and clinical view (anterior teeth: labial view; posterior teeth: mesial view)

Primary teeth have a whiter crown color, smaller overall size, prominent cervical ridge, and narrower roots. Permanent teeth have a yellower crown color, larger overall size, and wider roots.

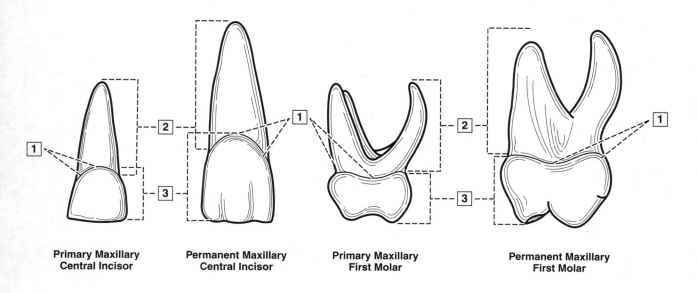

Primary Maxillary
Central Incisor

Permanent Maxillary
Central Incisor

Primary Maxillary
First Molar

Permanent Maxillary
First Molar

1 Cementoenamel junction

2 Root

3 Crown

NOTES

Copyright © 2008 by Saunders, an imprint of Elsevier Inc.

FIGURE 3-3 | Dental tissues and crown designations (anterior tooth: labiolingual section; posterior tooth: mesiodistal section)

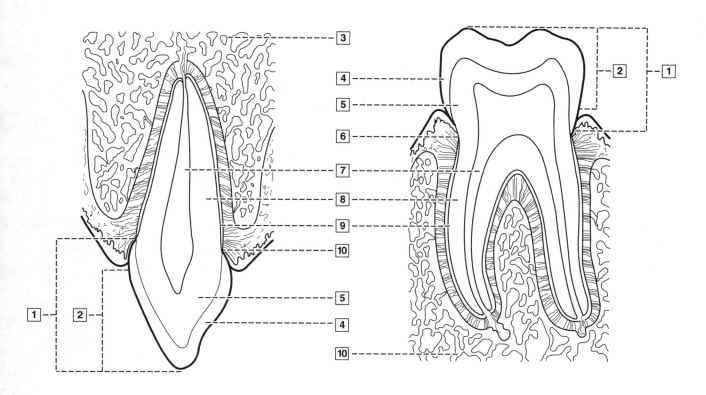

1	Anatomical crown	6	Cementoenamel junction
2	Clinical crown	7	Pulp cavity
3	Maxillary alveolar process	8	Dentin
4	Enamel	9	Cementum
5	Dentin	10	Mandibular alveolar process

Copyright © 2008 by Saunders, an imprint of Elsevier Inc.

NOTES

Copyright © 2008 by Saunders, an imprint of Elsevier Inc.

FIGURE 3-4 | Enamel (cross section and section along the length of the crystal with close-up views)

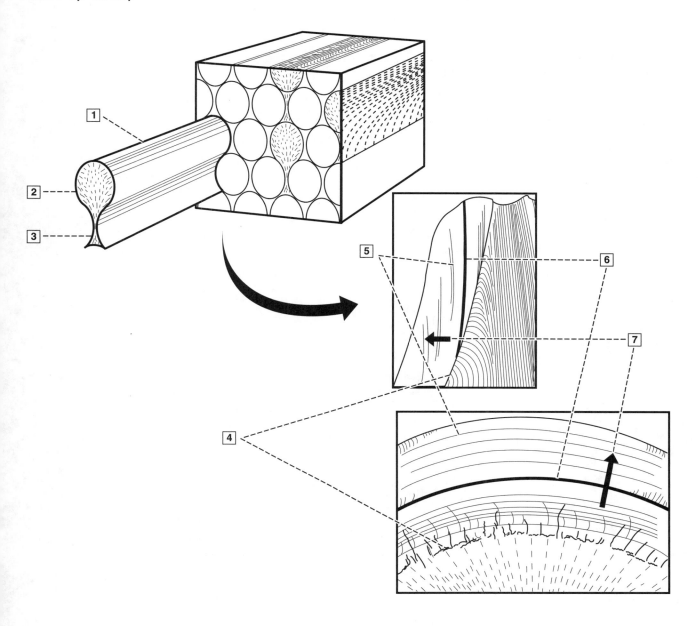

1 Enamel rod		**5** Lines of Retzius
2 Head portion		**6** Neonatal line
3 Tail portion		**7** Direction of enamel rod
4 Dentinoenamel junction		

Copyright © 2008 by Saunders, an imprint of Elsevier Inc.

NOTES

Copyright © 2008 by Saunders, an imprint of Elsevier Inc.

FIGURE 3-5 | Dentin (sagittal section with close-up view)

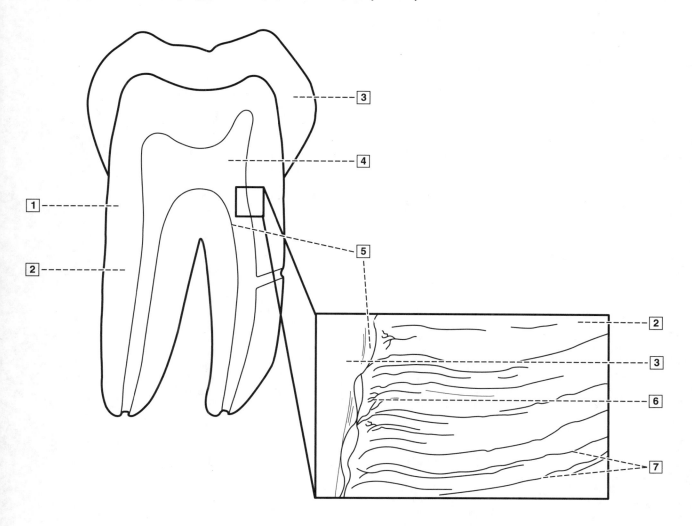

1 Mantle dentin   5 Dentinoenamel junction
2 Circumpulpal dentin   6 Odontoblastic processes
3 Enamel   7 Dentinal tubules
4 Pulp

Copyright © 2008 by Saunders, an imprint of Elsevier Inc.

NOTES

Copyright © 2008 by Saunders, an imprint of Elsevier Inc.

FIGURE 3-6 | Pulp in primary and permanent teeth (mesiodistal section)

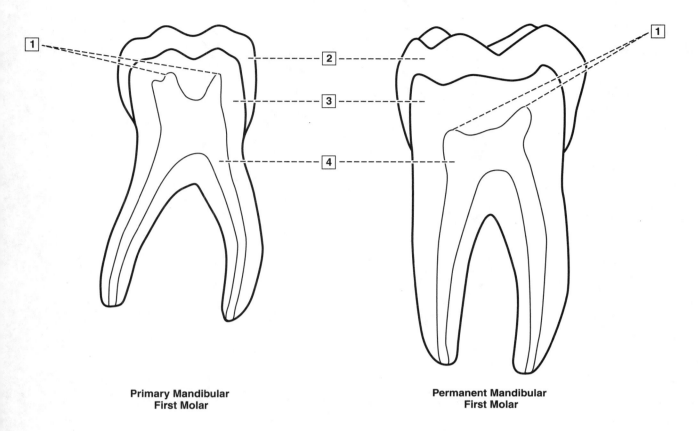

Primary Mandibular
First Molar

Permanent Mandibular
First Molar

1 Pulp horns

2 Enamel

3 Dentin

4 Pulp cavity

Copyright © 2008 by Saunders, an imprint of Elsevier Inc.

NOTES

Copyright © 2008 by Saunders, an imprint of Elsevier Inc.

FIGURE 3-7 | Pulp (mesiodistal section with close-up view)

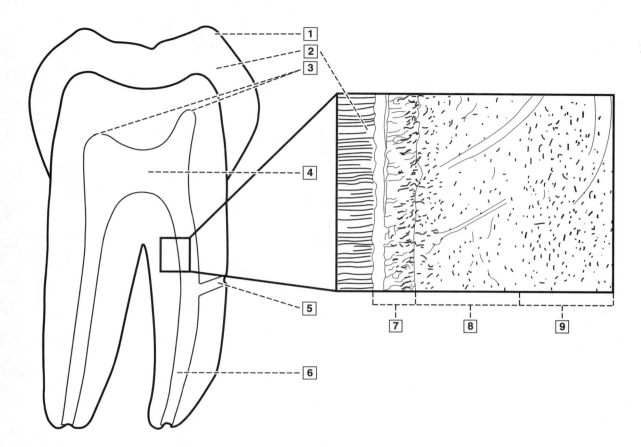

1 Enamel		**6** Radicular pulp
2 Dentin		**7** Odontoblastic layer
3 Pulp horns		**8** Cell-free zone
4 Coronal pulp		**9** Cell-rich zone
5 Accessory canal		

Copyright © 2008 by Saunders, an imprint of Elsevier Inc.

NOTES

Copyright © 2008 by Saunders, an imprint of Elsevier Inc.

FIGURE 3-8 | Periodontium (mesiodistal section)

Some dental anatomists include the gingival tissues as part of the periodontium.

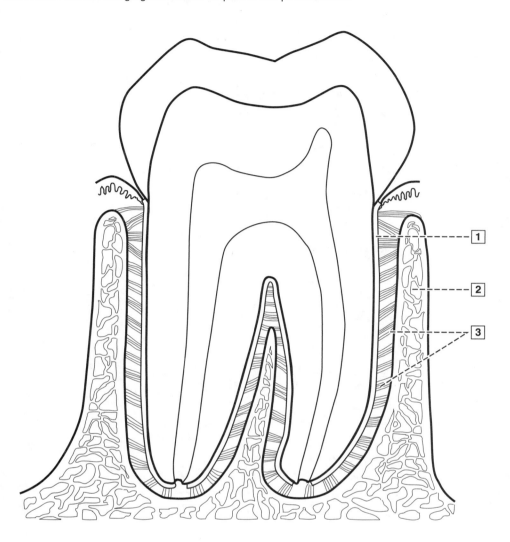

1 Cementum

2 Alveolar bone

3 Periodontal ligament

NOTES

Copyright © 2008 by Saunders, an imprint of Elsevier Inc.

FIGURE 3-9 | Dentin and cementum (close-up view)

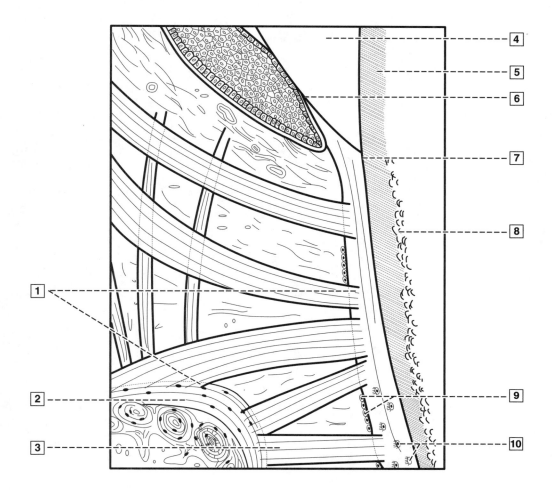

1	Sharpey's fibers	**6**	Cementoenamel junction
2	Alveolar crest of alveolar bone proper	**7**	Dentinocemental junction
3	Periodontal ligament	**8**	Tomes' granular layer in dentin
4	Enamel	**9**	Cementoblasts in pulp
5	Mantle dentin	**10**	Cementocytes in cementum

Copyright © 2008 by Saunders, an imprint of Elsevier Inc.

NOTES

Copyright © 2008 by Saunders, an imprint of Elsevier Inc.

FIGURE 3-10 | Alveolar bone (close-up view)

The alveolar crest has been slightly resorbed, which occurs even with a relatively healthy periodontium.

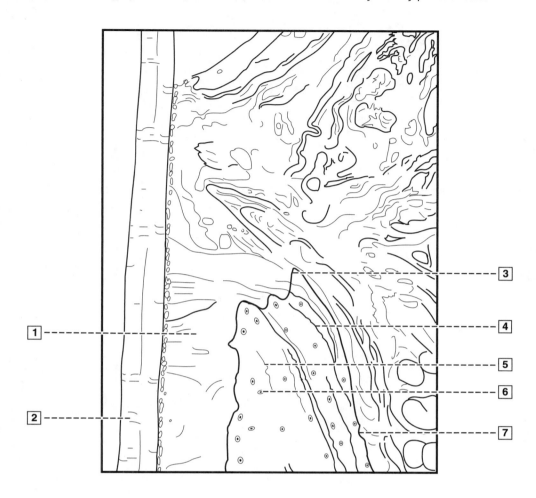

1	Periodontal ligament	5	Reversal line
2	Cementum	6	Osteocyte in lacuna
3	Alveolar crest	7	Howship's lacuna
4	Arrest line		

Copyright © 2008 by Saunders, an imprint of Elsevier Inc.

NOTES

Copyright © 2008 by Saunders, an imprint of Elsevier Inc.

FIGURE 3-11 | Periodontal ligament and alveolar bone (mesiodistal section)

Some dental researchers include the gingival fiber groups as part of the periodontal ligament. The interdental ligament is not shown in this view.

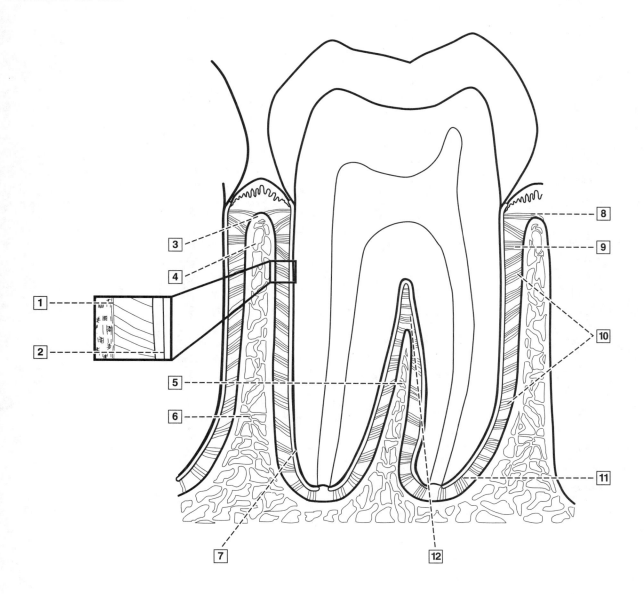

1	Sharpey's fibers within alveolar bone	7	Cementum
2	Sharpey's fibers within cementum	8	Alveolar crest group
3	Alveolar crest	9	Horizontal group
4	Alveolar bone	10	Oblique group
5	Interradicular septum	11	Apical group
6	Interdental bone	12	Interradicular group

Copyright © 2008 by Saunders, an imprint of Elsevier Inc.

NOTES

Copyright © 2008 by Saunders, an imprint of Elsevier Inc.

FIGURE 3-12 | Interdental ligament (anterior view and mesiodistal section)

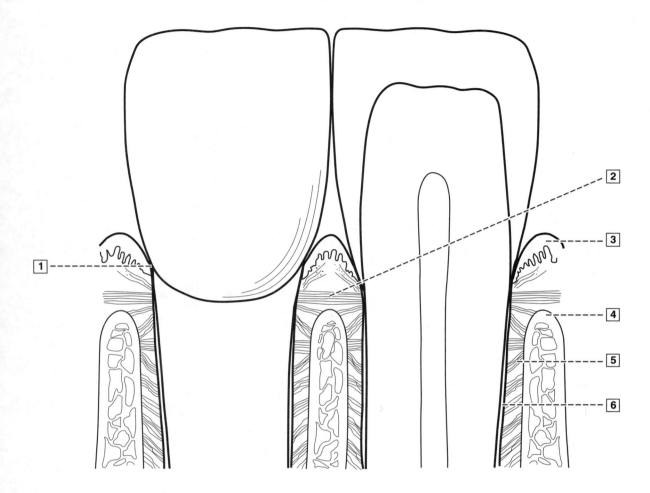

1 Cementoenamel junction

2 Interdental ligament

3 Interdental papilla

4 Alveolar crest

5 Alveolodental fibers

6 Cementum

Copyright © 2008 by Saunders, an imprint of Elsevier Inc.

NOTES

Copyright © 2008 by Saunders, an imprint of Elsevier Inc.

FIGURE 3-13 | Gingival fiber group (frontal view and labiolingual section)

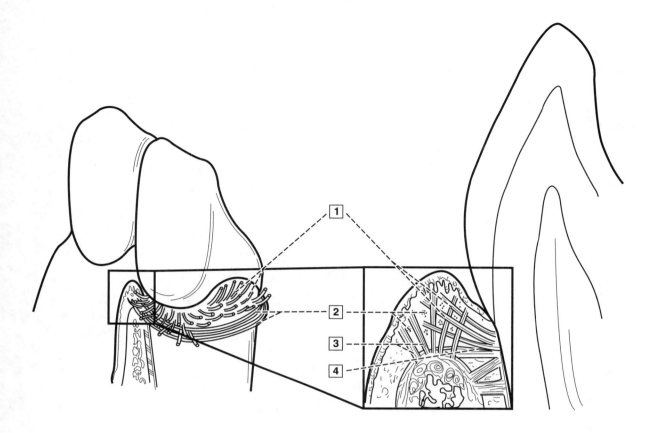

[1] Dentogingival ligament
[2] Circular ligament
[3] Alveologingival ligament
[4] Dentoperiosteal ligament

Copyright © 2008 by Saunders, an imprint of Elsevier Inc.

NOTES

Copyright © 2008 by Saunders, an imprint of Elsevier Inc.

FIGURE 3-14 | Primary dentitions (occlusal views)

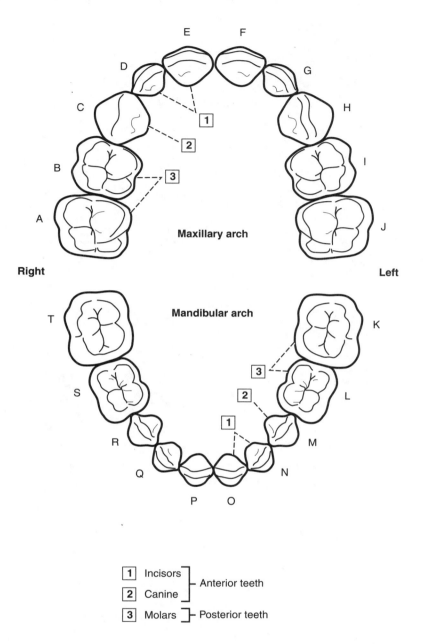

Maxillary arch

Right   Left

Mandibular arch

1 Incisors ⎫
           ⎬ Anterior teeth
2 Canine ⎭

3 Molars ⎤ Posterior teeth

Copyright © 2008 by Saunders, an imprint of Elsevier Inc.

NOTES

Copyright © 2008 by Saunders, an imprint of Elsevier Inc.

FIGURE 3-15 | Permanent dentitions (occlusal views)

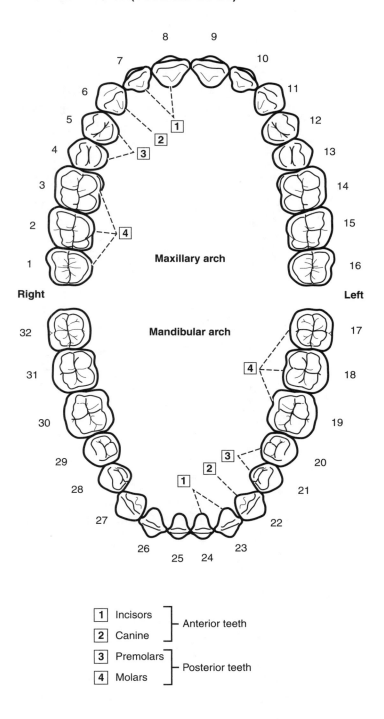

1 Incisors ⎤
2 Canine ⎦ — Anterior teeth

3 Premolars ⎤
4 Molars ⎦ — Posterior teeth

Copyright © 2008 by Saunders, an imprint of Elsevier Inc.

NOTES

Copyright © 2008 by Saunders, an imprint of Elsevier Inc.

FIGURE 3-16 | Surfaces of the teeth and their orientational relationship to other oral cavity structures, to the midline, and to other teeth

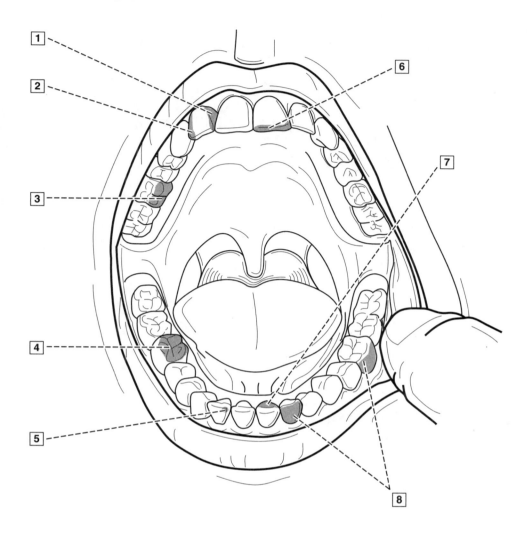

1 Mesial surface		**5** Proximal surface with contact area
2 Distal surface		**6** Incisal surface
3 Palatal surface		**7** Lingual surface
4 Occlusal surface		**8** Facial surfaces: labial and buccal surfaces

Copyright © 2008 by Saunders, an imprint of Elsevier Inc.

NOTES

Copyright © 2008 by Saunders, an imprint of Elsevier Inc.

FIGURE 3-17 │ Maxillary right central incisor (lingual and incisal views)

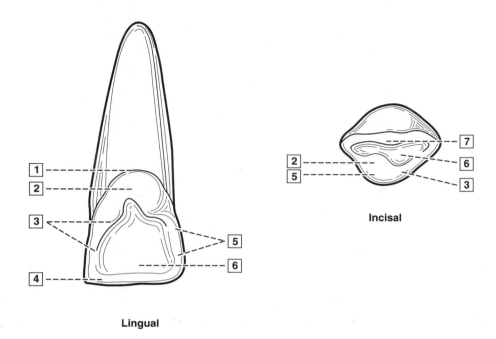

Lingual

Incisal

1	Cementoenamel junction
2	Cingulum
3	Mesial marginal ridge
4	Linguoincisal edge
5	Distal marginal ridge
6	Lingual fossa
7	Incisal ridge

NOTES

Copyright © 2008 by Saunders, an imprint of Elsevier Inc.

FIGURE 3-18 | Maxillary right lateral incisor (lingual and incisal views)

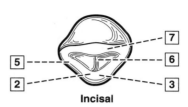

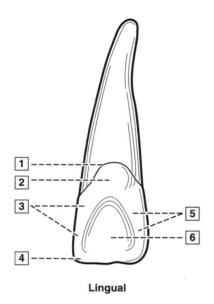

Incisal

Lingual

1	Cementoenamel junction
2	Cingulum
3	Mesial marginal ridge
4	Linguoincisal edge
5	Distal marginal ridge
6	Lingual fossa
7	Incisal ridge

NOTES

Copyright © 2008 by Saunders, an imprint of Elsevier Inc.

FIGURE 3-19 | Mandibular right central incisor (lingual and incisal views)

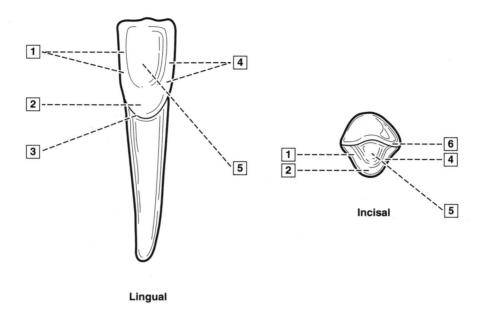

Lingual

Incisal

1	Mesial marginal ridge
2	Cingulum
3	Cementoenamel junction
4	Distal marginal ridge
5	Lingual fossa
6	Incisal ridge

Copyright © 2008 by Saunders, an imprint of Elsevier Inc.

NOTES

Copyright © 2008 by Saunders, an imprint of Elsevier Inc.

FIGURE 3-20 | Mandibular right lateral incisor (lingual and incisal views)

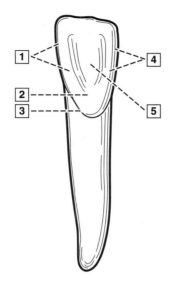

Lingual

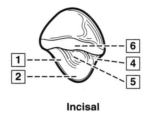

Incisal

1 Mesial marginal ridge

2 Cingulum

3 Cementoenamel junction

4 Distal marginal ridge

5 Lingual fossa

6 Incisal ridge

Copyright © 2008 by Saunders, an imprint of Elsevier Inc.

NOTES

Copyright © 2008 by Saunders, an imprint of Elsevier Inc.

FIGURE 3-21 | Maxillary right canine (lingual and incisal views)

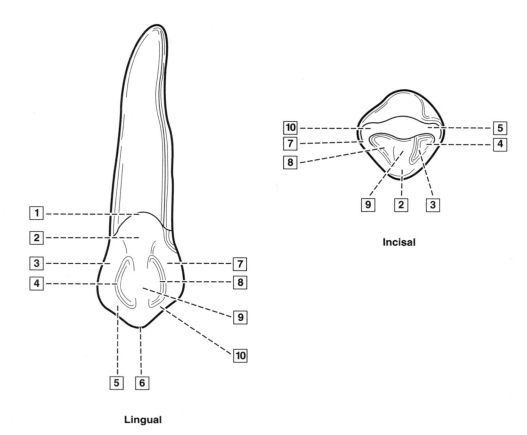

Incisal

Lingual

1	Cementoenamel junction		6	Cusp tip
2	Cingulum		7	Distal marginal ridge
3	Mesial marginal ridge		8	Distolingual fossa
4	Mesiolingual fossa		9	Lingual ridge
5	Mesial cusp ridge		10	Distal cusp ridge

Copyright © 2008 by Saunders, an imprint of Elsevier Inc.

NOTES

Copyright © 2008 by Saunders, an imprint of Elsevier Inc.

FIGURE 3-22 | Mandibular right canine (lingual and incisal views)

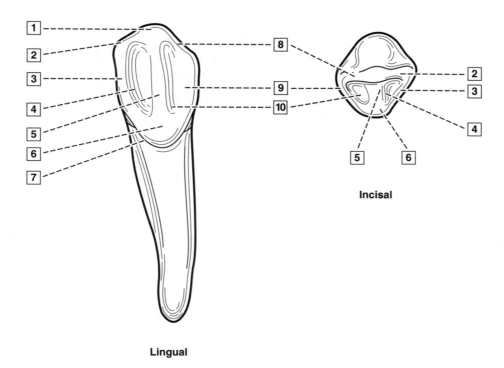

Incisal

Lingual

1	Cusp tip	6	Cingulum
2	Mesial cusp ridge	7	Cementoenamel junction
3	Mesial marginal ridge	8	Distal cusp ridge
4	Mesiolingual fossa	9	Distal marginal ridge
5	Lingual ridge	10	Distolingual fossa

NOTES

Copyright © 2008 by Saunders, an imprint of Elsevier Inc.

FIGURE 3-23 | Maxillary right first premolar (mesial and occlusal views)

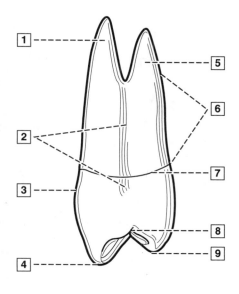

Mesial

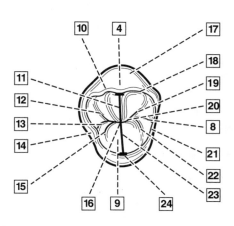

Occlusal

1	Buccal root
2	Mesial developmental depression
3	Buccal cervical ridge
4	Buccal cusp
5	Lingual root
6	Root trunk
7	Cementoenamel junction
8	Mesial marginal groove
9	Lingual cusp
10	Distal cusp ridge of buccal cusp

11	Lingual cusp ridge of buccal cusp (buccal triangular ridge)
12	Distobuccal triangular groove
13	Distal triangular fossa (with distal pit)
14	Distal marginal ridge
15	Distolingual triangular groove
16	Central groove
17	Buccal cusp ridge of the buccal cusp
18	Mesial cusp ridge of the buccal cusp

19	Mesiobuccal triangular groove
20	Mesial triangular fossa (with mesial pit)
21	Mesial marginal ridge
22	Mesiolingual triangular groove
23	Lingual triangular ridge
24	Transverse ridge

Copyright © 2008 by Saunders, an imprint of Elsevier Inc.

NOTES

Copyright © 2008 by Saunders, an imprint of Elsevier Inc.

FIGURE 3-24 | Maxillary right second premolar (mesial and occlusal views)

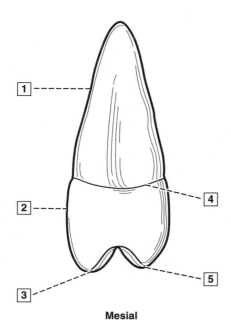

Mesial

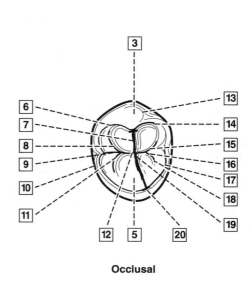

Occlusal

1 Root	**8** Distobuccal triangular groove	**15** Mesiobuccal triangular groove
2 Buccal cervical ridge	**9** Distal triangular fossa (with distal pit)	**16** Mesial triangular fossa (with mesial pit)
3 Buccal cusp	**10** Distal marginal ridge	**17** Mesial marginal ridge
4 Cementoenamel junction	**11** Distolingual triangular groove	**18** Mesiolingual triangular groove
5 Lingual cusp	**12** Central groove	**19** Lingual triangular ridge
6 Distal cusp ridge of buccal cusp	**13** Buccal cusp ridge of the buccal cusp	**20** Transverse ridge
7 Lingual cusp ridge of buccal cusp (buccal triangular ridge)	**14** Mesial cusp ridge of the buccal cusp	

NOTES

Copyright © 2008 by Saunders, an imprint of Elsevier Inc.

FIGURE 3-25 | Mandibular right first premolar (mesial and occlusal views)

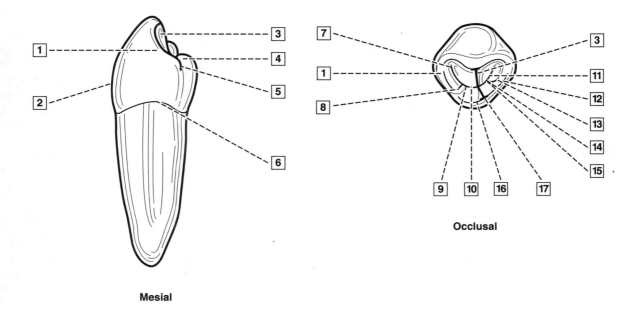

Mesial

Occlusal

1	Mesial marginal ridge	10	Central groove
2	Buccal cervical ridge	11	Distobuccal triangular groove
3	Buccal triangular ridge	12	Distal marginal ridge
4	Lingual cusp	13	Distal marginal groove
5	Mesiolingual groove	14	Distolingual triangular groove
6	Cementoenamel junction	15	Distal fossa (with distal pit)
7	Mesiobuccal triangular groove	16	Lingual triangular ridge
8	Mesiolingual groove	17	Transverse ridge
9	Mesial fossa (with mesial pit)		

Copyright © 2008 by Saunders, an imprint of Elsevier Inc.

NOTES

Copyright © 2008 by Saunders, an imprint of Elsevier Inc.

FIGURE 3-26 ∣ Mandibular right second premolar (mesial and occlusal views of the three-cusp type)

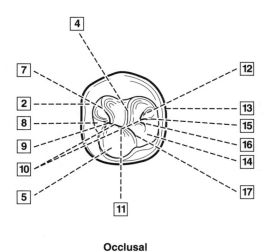

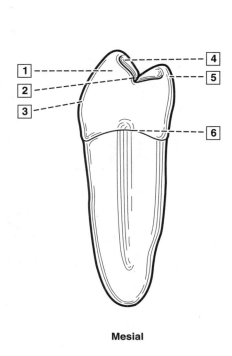

Mesial

Occlusal

1	Buccal cusp		10	Central groove
2	Mesial marginal ridge		11	Central pit
3	Buccal cervical ridge		12	Distobuccal triangular groove
4	Buccal triangular ridge		13	Distal marginal ridge
5	Mesiolingual cusp		14	Distolingual cusp
6	Cementoenamel junction		15	Distal marginal groove
7	Mesiobuccal triangular groove		16	Distal fossa (with distal pit)
8	Mesial marginal groove		17	Lingual groove
9	Mesial fossa (with mesial pit)			

Copyright © 2008 by Saunders, an imprint of Elsevier Inc.

NOTES

Copyright © 2008 by Saunders, an imprint of Elsevier Inc.

FIGURE 3-27 | Maxillary right first molar (lingual, mesial, and occlusal views)

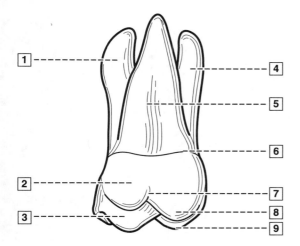

Lingual

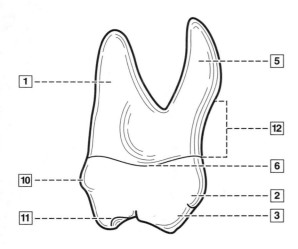

Mesial

Occlusal

[1]	Mesiobuccal root
[2]	Cusp of Carabelli
[3]	Mesiolingual cusp
[4]	Distobuccal root
[5]	Lingual root
[6]	Cementoenamel junction
[7]	Distolingual groove
[8]	Distolingual cusp
[9]	Distobuccal cusp
[10]	Cervical ridge
[11]	Mesiobuccal cusp
[12]	Root trunk
[13]	Buccal groove
[14]	Distal marginal ridge
[15]	Distal marginal ridge groove
[16]	Distal fossa with distal pit
[17]	Distolingual cusp ridge
[18]	Distal fossa (with distal pit)
[19]	Distolingual cusp ridge
[20]	Oblique ridge
[21]	Mesiobuccal cusp ridge
[22]	Mesiobuccal triangular groove
[23]	Mesial marginal ridge
[24]	Mesial fossa (with mesial pit)
[25]	Mesial marginal ridge groove
[26]	Transverse ridge
[27]	Mesiolingual triangular groove
[28]	Mesiolingual cusp ridge
[29]	Central groove with central pit

Copyright © 2008 by Saunders, an imprint of Elsevier Inc.

NOTES

Copyright © 2008 by Saunders, an imprint of Elsevier Inc.

FIGURE 3-28 | Maxillary right second molar—rhomboidal crown outline (lingual, mesial, and occlusal views)

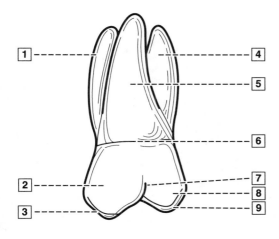

Lingual

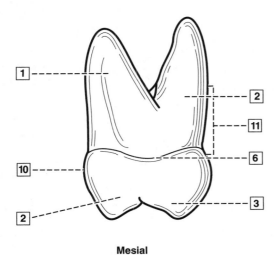

Mesial

Occlusal

1. Mesiobuccal root
2. Mesiolingual cusp
3. Mesiobuccal cusp
4. Distobuccal root
5. Lingual root
6. Cementoenamel junction
7. Distolingual groove
8. Distolingual cusp
9. Distobuccal cusp
10. Cervical ridge
11. Root trunk
12. Buccal groove
13. Distobuccal cusp ridge
14. Distobuccal triangular groove
15. Distal marginal ridge
16. Distal marginal ridge groove
17. Distal fossa (with distal pit)
18. Distolingual cusp ridge
19. Oblique ridge
20. Mesiobuccal cusp ridge
21. Mesiobuccal triangular groove
22. Mesial marginal ridge
23. Mesial marginal ridge groove
24. Mesial fossa (with mesial pit)
25. Mesiolingual cusp ridge
26. Mesiolingual triangular groove
27. Transverse ridge
28. Central groove with central pit

NOTES

Copyright © 2008 by Saunders, an imprint of Elsevier Inc.

FIGURE 3-29 | Mandibular right first molar (lingual, mesial, and occlusal views)

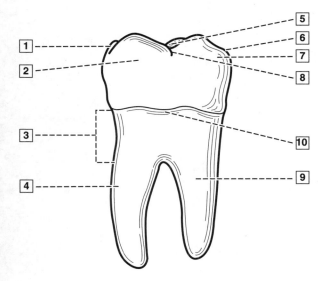

Lingual

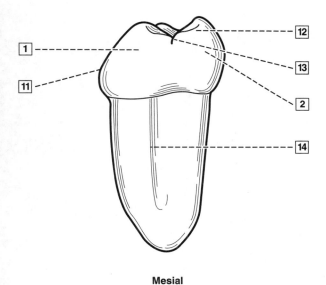

Mesial

Occlusal

1	Mesiobuccal cusp
2	Mesiolingual cusp
3	Root trunk
4	Mesial root
5	Distobuccal cusp
6	Distal cusp
7	Distolingual cusp
8	Lingual groove
9	Distal root
10	Cementoenamel junction
11	Cervical ridge
12	Mesial marginal ridge
13	Mesial marginal ridge groove
14	Mesial fluting
15	Mesiobuccal groove
16	Mesiobuccal cusp ridge
17	Mesial triangular fossa (with mesial pit)
18	Mesiolingual cusp ridge
19	Distobuccal cusp ridge
20	Distobuccal groove
21	Distal cusp ridge
22	Distal marginal ridge
23	Distal marginal ridge groove
24	Distal triangular fossa (with distal pit)
25	Distolingual cusp ridge
26	Central groove with central pit

Copyright © 2008 by Saunders, an imprint of Elsevier Inc.

NOTES

 Copyright © 2008 by Saunders, an imprint of Elsevier Inc.

FIGURE 3-30 | Mandibular right second molar (lingual, mesial, and occlusal views)

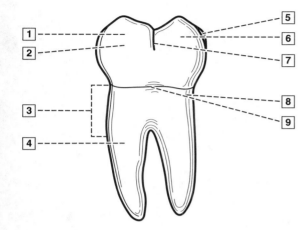

Lingual

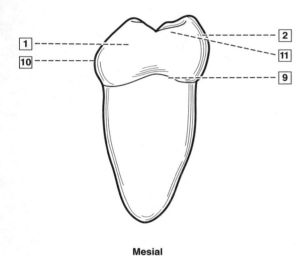

Mesial

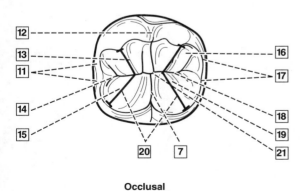

Occlusal

1 Mesiobuccal cusp
2 Mesiolingual cusp
3 Root trunk
4 Mesial root
5 Distobuccal cusp
6 Distolingual cusp
7 Lingual groove
8 Distal root
9 Cementoenamel junction
10 Cervical ridge
11 Mesial marginal ridge
12 Buccal groove
13 Mesiobuccal cusp ridge
14 Mesial triangular fossa (with mesial pit)
15 Mesiolingual cusp ridge
16 Distobuccal cusp ridge
17 Distal marginal ridge
18 Distal triangular fossa (with distal pit)
19 Distolingual cusp ridge
20 Transverse ridges
21 Central groove with central pit

NOTES

Copyright © 2008 by Saunders, an imprint of Elsevier Inc.

FIGURE 4-1 | Skull bones (frontal view)

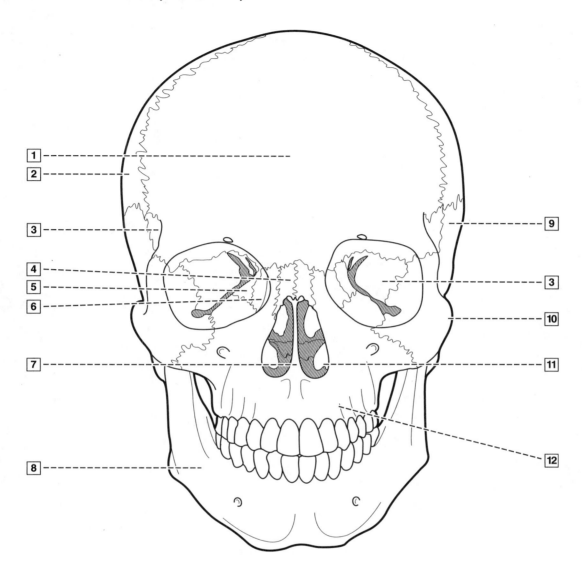

1	Frontal bone	7	Vomer bone
2	Parietal bone	8	Mandible
3	Sphenoid bone	9	Temporal bone
4	Nasal bone	10	Zygomatic bone
5	Ethmoid bone	11	Inferior nasal concha
6	Lacrimal bone	12	Maxilla

Copyright © 2008 by Saunders, an imprint of Elsevier Inc.

NOTES

Copyright © 2008 by Saunders, an imprint of Elsevier Inc.

FIGURE 4-2 | Skull bones and landmarks (lateral view)

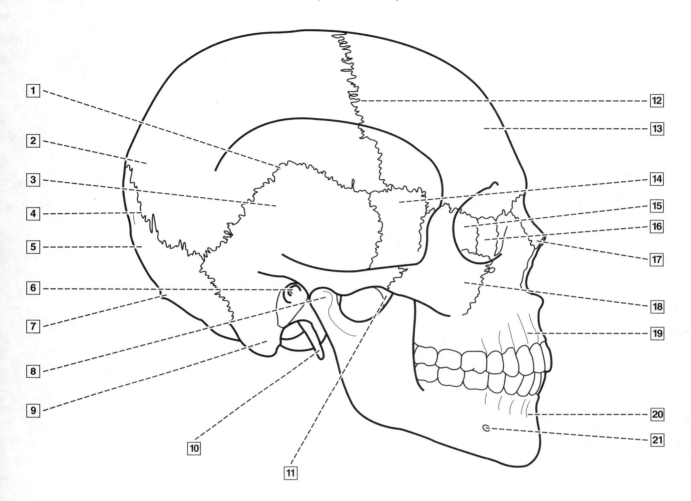

1	Squamosal suture	8	Condyloid process	15	Ethmoid bone
2	Parietal bone	9	Mastoid process of temporal bone	16	Lacrimal bone
3	Temporal bone	10	Styloid process	17	Nasal bone
4	Lambdoidal suture	11	Pterygoid process	18	Zygomatic bone
5	Occipital bone	12	Coronal suture	19	Maxilla
6	External auditory meatus	13	Frontal bone	20	Mandible
7	External occipital protuberance	14	Sphenoid bone	21	Mental foramen

Copyright © 2008 by Saunders, an imprint of Elsevier Inc.

NOTES

Copyright © 2008 by Saunders, an imprint of Elsevier Inc.

FIGURE 4-3 ❘ Skull bones and landmarks (inferior view)

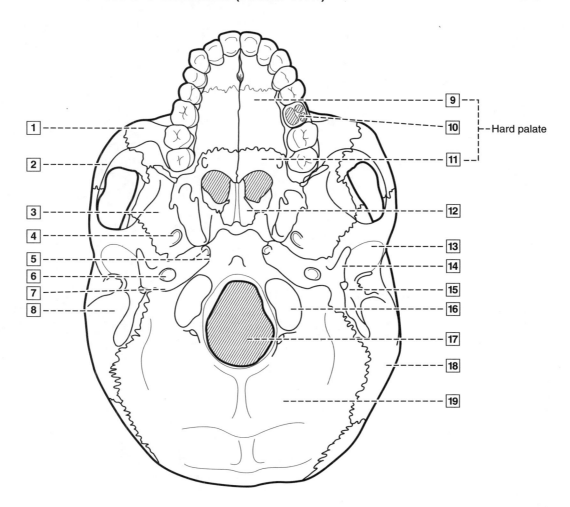

1 Zygomatic process of maxilla	**8** Mastoid process	**15** Stylomastoid foramen
2 Zygomatic bone	**9** Maxilla (palatine process)	**16** Occipital condyle
3 Sphenoid bone	**10** Alveolar process	**17** Foramen magnum
4 Foramen ovale	**11** Palatine bone (horizontal plate)	**18** Temporal bone
5 Foramen lacerum	**12** Vomer bone	**19** Occipital bone
6 Carotid canal	**13** Mandibular fossa	
7 Jugular foramen	**14** Styloid process	

Copyright © 2008 by Saunders, an imprint of Elsevier Inc.

NOTES

Copyright © 2008 by Saunders, an imprint of Elsevier Inc.

FIGURE 4-4 | Skull bones and landmarks (internal view)

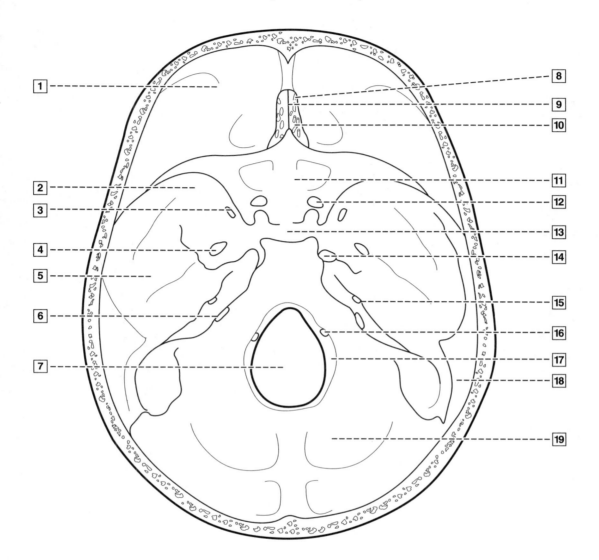

1 Frontal bone	8 Ethmoid bone	15 Internal auditory meatus
2 Greater wing of sphenoid	9 Crista galli	16 Hypoglossal canal
3 Foramen rotundum	10 Cribriform plate	17 Hypoglossal foramen
4 Foramen ovale	11 Sphenoid bone	18 Parietal bone
5 Temporal bone	12 Optic foramen	19 Occipital bone
6 Jugular foramen	13 Sella turcica	
7 Foramen magnum	14 Foramen lacerum	

Copyright © 2008 by Saunders, an imprint of Elsevier Inc.

NOTES

Copyright © 2008 by Saunders, an imprint of Elsevier Inc.

FIGURE 4-5 | Skull bones and landmarks (midsagittal section)

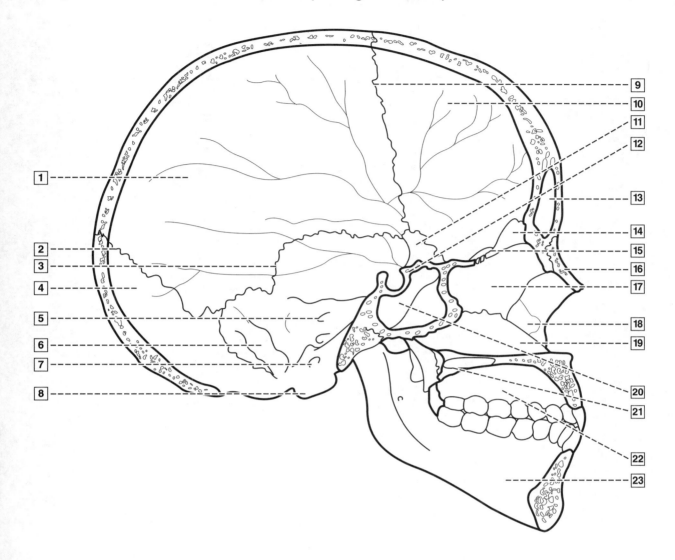

1 Parietal bone	**9** Coronal suture	**17** Ethmoid bone (perpendicular plate)
2 Lambdoidal suture	**10** Frontal bone	**18** Inferior nasal concha
3 Squamosal suture	**11** Sphenoid bone	**19** Vomer bone
4 Occipital bone	**12** Sella turcica	**20** Sphenoidal sinus
5 Internal auditory meatus	**13** Frontal sinus	**21** Palatine bone
6 Temporal bone	**14** Crista galli of ethmoid	**22** Maxilla
7 Hypoglossal canal	**15** Cribriform plate	**23** Mandible
8 Occipital condyle	**16** Nasal bone	

Copyright © 2008 by Saunders, an imprint of Elsevier Inc.

NOTES

Copyright © 2008 by Saunders, an imprint of Elsevier Inc.

FIGURE 4-6 | Maxilla and landmarks (anterior view)

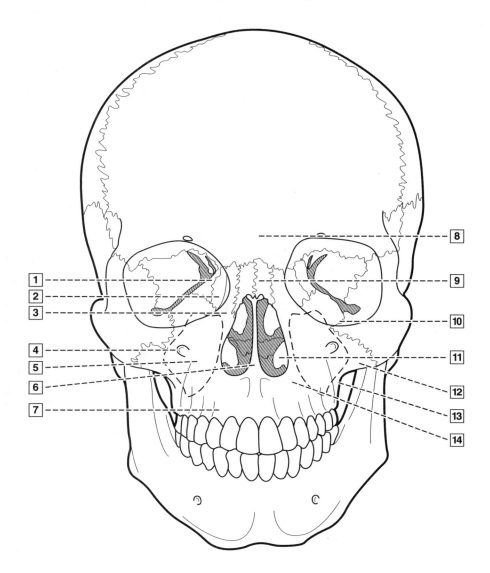

1	Ethmoid bone	**6**	Vomer	**11**	Inferior nasal concha
2	Lacrimal bone	**7**	Alveolar process of maxilla	**12**	Zygomatic process of maxilla
3	Frontal process of maxilla	**8**	Frontal bone	**13**	Location of maxillary sinus
4	Infraorbital foramen	**9**	Nasal bone	**14**	Canine fossa
5	Body of maxilla	**10**	Infraorbital sulcus		

Copyright © 2008 by Saunders, an imprint of Elsevier Inc.

NOTES

Copyright © 2008 by Saunders, an imprint of Elsevier Inc.

FIGURE 4-7 | Maxilla and landmarks (cutaway lateral aspect)

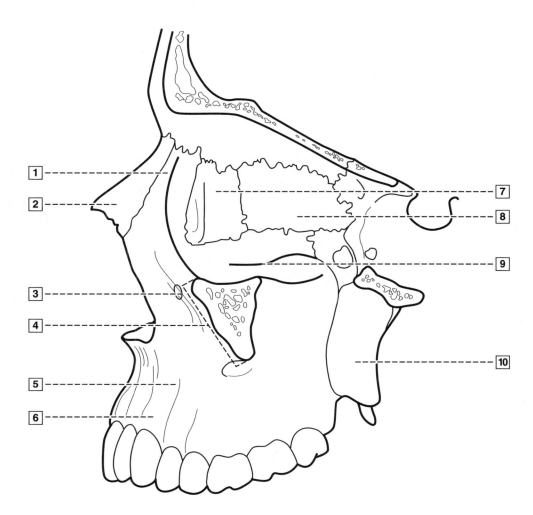

1	Frontal process of maxilla	6	Canine eminence
2	Nasal bone	7	Lacrimal bone
3	Infraorbital foramen	8	Ethmoid bone
4	Zygomatic process of maxilla	9	Infraorbital sulcus
5	Canine fossa	10	Sphenoid bone

Copyright © 2008 by Saunders, an imprint of Elsevier Inc.

NOTES

Copyright © 2008 by Saunders, an imprint of Elsevier Inc.

FIGURE 4-8 | Mandible and landmarks (lateral view)

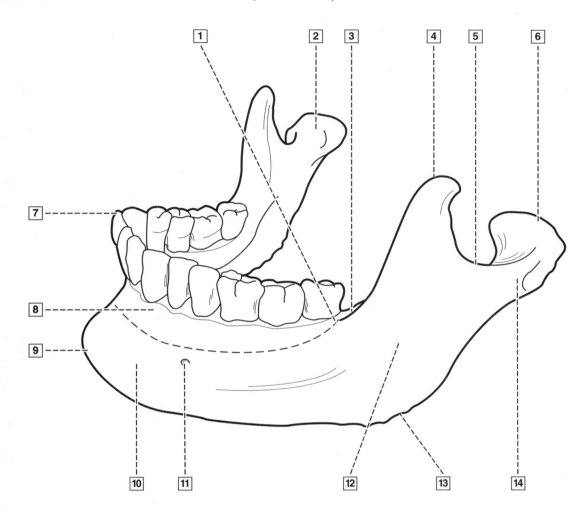

1 External oblique line	**6** Articulating surface of condyle	**11** Mental foramen
2 Pterygoid fovea	**7** Mandibular teeth	**12** Ramus
3 Coronoid notch	**8** Alveolar process	**13** Angle
4 Coronoid process	**9** Mental protuberance	**14** Neck
5 Mandibular notch	**10** Body	

Copyright © 2008 by Saunders, an imprint of Elsevier Inc.

NOTES

Copyright © 2008 by Saunders, an imprint of Elsevier Inc.

FIGURE 4-9 | Mandible and landmarks (medial view)

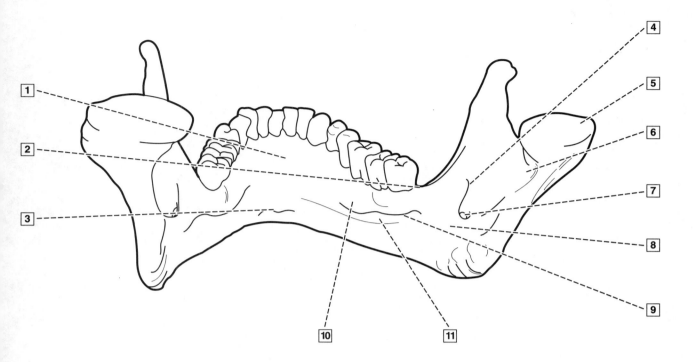

1	Alveolar process	7	Mandibular foramen
2	Retromolar triangle	8	Mylohyoid groove
3	Genial tubercles	9	Mylohyoid line
4	Lingula	10	Sublingual fossa
5	Articulating surface of condyle	11	Submandibular fossa
6	Ramus		

Copyright © 2008 by Saunders, an imprint of Elsevier Inc.

NOTES

Copyright © 2008 by Saunders, an imprint of Elsevier Inc.

FIGURE 4-10 | Orbit (anterior view)

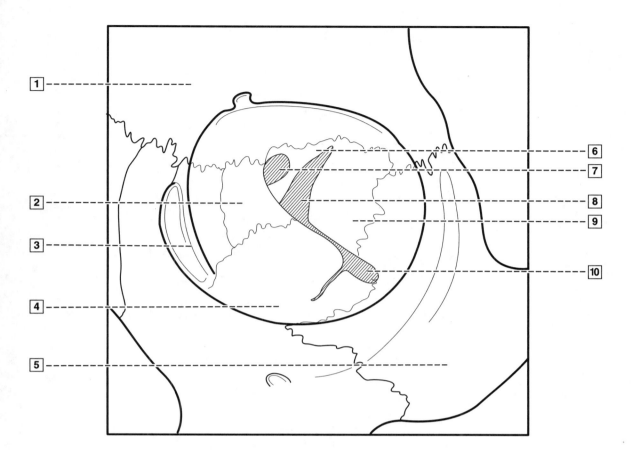

1	Frontal bone	6	Lesser wing of sphenoid bone
2	Ethmoid bone	7	Optic canal
3	Lacrimal bone	8	Superior orbital fissure
4	Maxilla	9	Greater wing of sphenoid bone
5	Zygomatic bone	10	Inferior orbital fissure

NOTES

Copyright © 2008 by Saunders, an imprint of Elsevier Inc.

FIGURE 4-11 | Nasal region (anterior view)

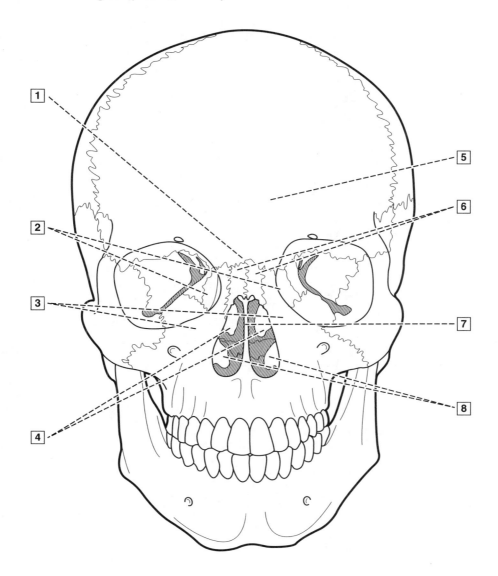

1	Nasion	**5**	Frontal bone
2	Lacrimal bones	**6**	Nasal bones
3	Maxillae	**7**	Nasal septum
4	Middle nasal conchae	**8**	Inferior nasal conchae

Copyright © 2008 by Saunders, an imprint of Elsevier Inc.

NOTES

Copyright © 2008 by Saunders, an imprint of Elsevier Inc.

FIGURE 4-12 ∣ Nasal cavity (sagittal section of the lateral wall)

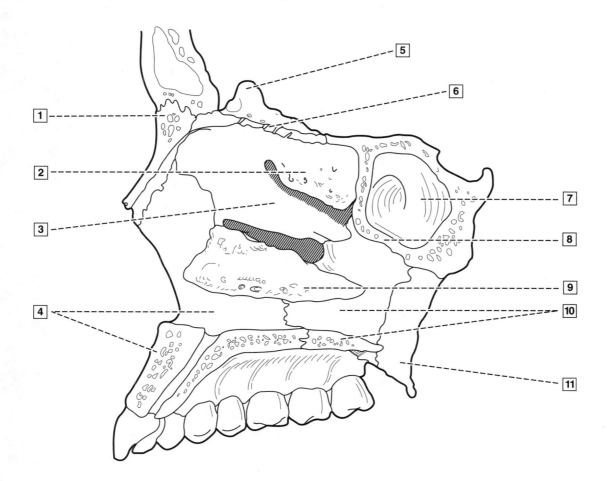

1	Nasal bone	7	Sphenoidal sinus
2	Superior nasal concha	8	Sphenoid bone
3	Middle nasal concha	9	Inferior nasal concha
4	Maxilla	10	Palatine bone
5	Crista galli	11	Medial pterygoid plate
6	Cribriform plate		

Copyright © 2008 by Saunders, an imprint of Elsevier Inc.

NOTES

Copyright © 2008 by Saunders, an imprint of Elsevier Inc.

FIGURE 4-13 | Nasal cavity (sagittal section of the medial wall)

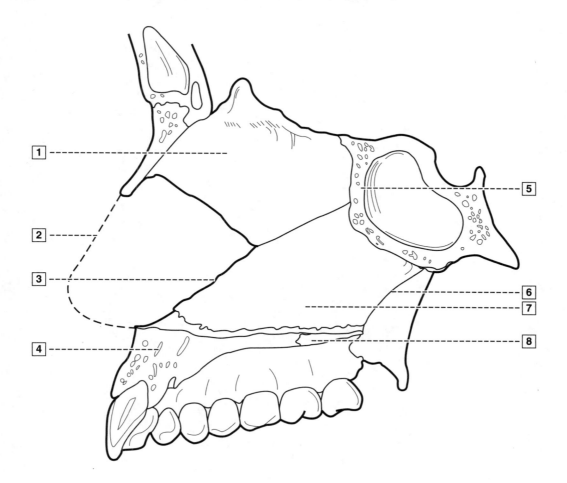

1 Ethmoid bone		**5** Sphenoid bone
2 Outline of nasal cartilage		**6** Free border
3 Articulation with nasal cartilage		**7** Vomer
4 Maxilla		**8** Palatine bone

NOTES

Copyright © 2008 by Saunders, an imprint of Elsevier Inc.

FIGURE 4-14 | Zygomatic arch (lateral view)

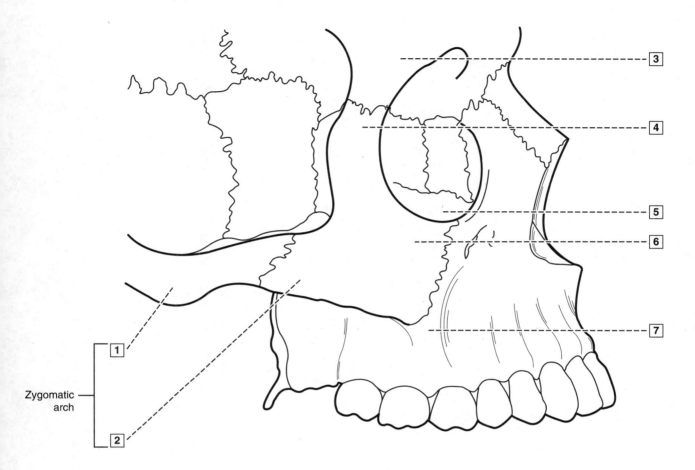

1 Zygomatic process of temporal bone
2 Temporal process of zygomatic bone
3 Zygomatic process of frontal bone
4 Frontal process of zygomatic bone

5 Infraorbital rim
6 Maxillary process of zygomatic bone
7 Zygomatic process of maxillary bone

Copyright © 2008 by Saunders, an imprint of Elsevier Inc.

NOTES

Copyright © 2008 by Saunders, an imprint of Elsevier Inc.

FIGURE 4-15 | Temporomandibular joint (lateral view)

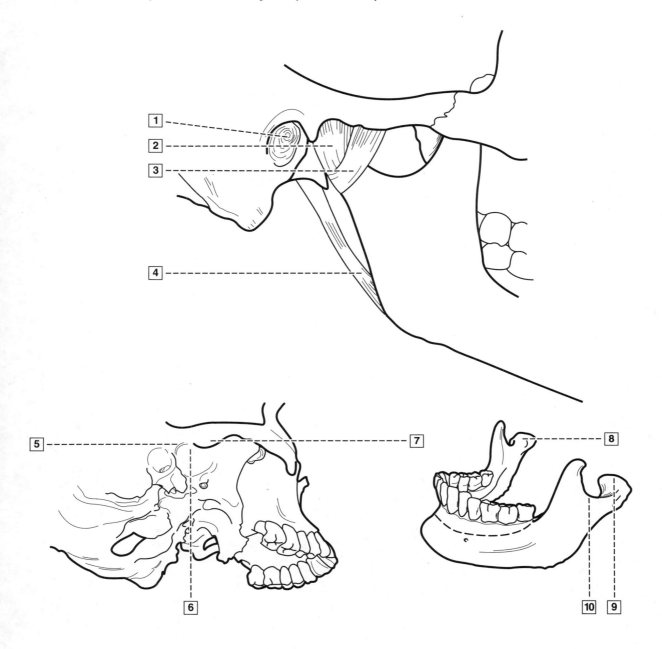

1	External acoustic meatus	6	Articular fossa
2	Joint capsule	7	Articular eminence
3	Temporomandibular ligament	8	Articulating surface of condyle
4	Stylomandibular ligament	9	Condyle of mandible
5	Postglenoid process	10	Mandibular notch

Copyright © 2008 by Saunders, an imprint of Elsevier Inc.

NOTES

Copyright © 2008 by Saunders, an imprint of Elsevier Inc.

FIGURE 4-16 | Temporomandibular joint (internal view)

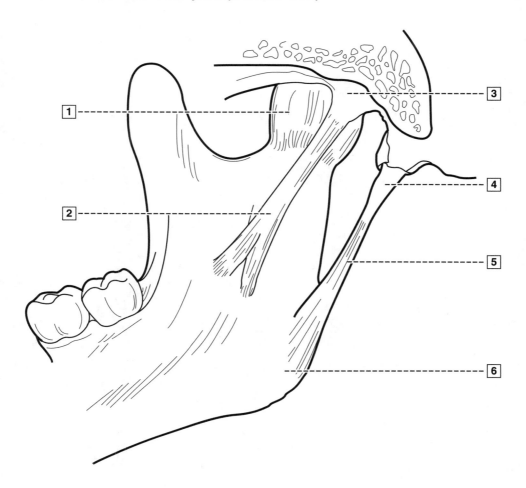

1 Joint capsule
2 Sphenomandibular ligament
3 Spine of sphenoid bone
4 Styloid process of temporal bone
5 Stylomandibular ligament
6 Angle of mandible

Copyright © 2008 by Saunders, an imprint of Elsevier Inc.

NOTES

Copyright © 2008 by Saunders, an imprint of Elsevier Inc.

FIGURE 4-17 | Temporomandibular joint (sagittal section with capsule removed)

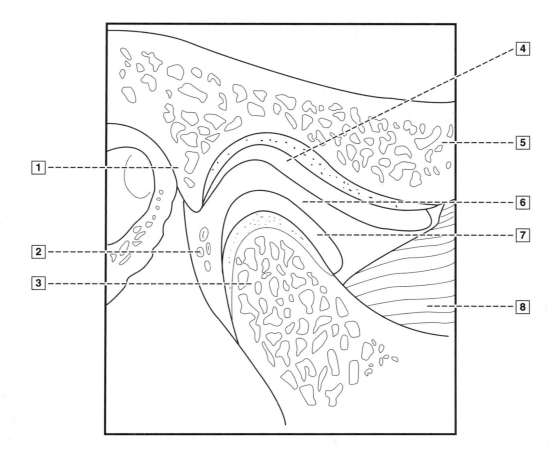

1	Postglenoid process	**5**	Articular eminence
2	Blood vessels	**6**	Joint disc
3	Condyle	**7**	Lower synovial cavity
4	Upper synovial cavity	**8**	Lateral pterygoid muscle

Copyright © 2008 by Saunders, an imprint of Elsevier Inc.

NOTES

Copyright © 2008 by Saunders, an imprint of Elsevier Inc.

FIGURE 4-18 | Hard palate (inferior view)

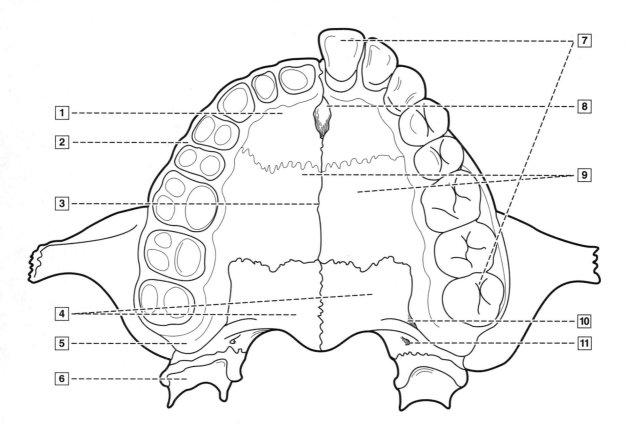

1	Palatine process of the maxilla	**7**	Maxillary teeth
2	Alveolar process of maxilla	**8**	Incisive foramen
3	Median palatine suture	**9**	Maxillae
4	Palatine bones	**10**	Greater palatine foramen
5	Maxillary tuberosity	**11**	Lesser palatine foramen
6	Sphenoid bone		

Copyright © 2008 by Saunders, an imprint of Elsevier Inc.

NOTES

Copyright © 2008 by Saunders, an imprint of Elsevier Inc.

FIGURE 4-19 | Paranasal sinuses (anterior aspect)

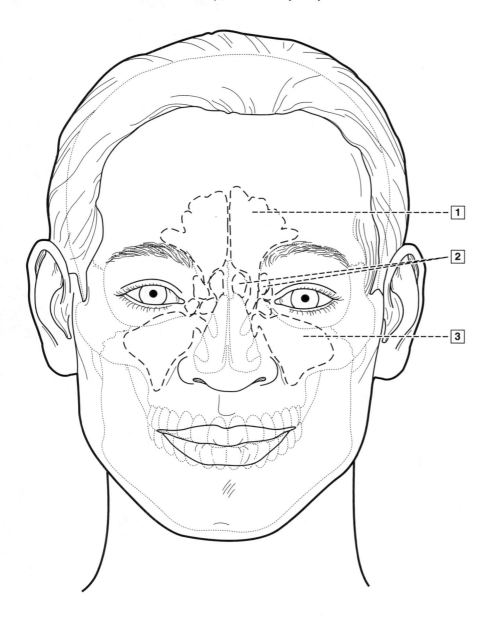

1 Frontal sinus
2 Ethmoidal sinuses
3 Maxillary sinus

Copyright © 2008 by Saunders, an imprint of Elsevier Inc.

NOTES

Copyright © 2008 by Saunders, an imprint of Elsevier Inc.

FIGURE 4-20 | Paranasal sinuses (lateral aspect)

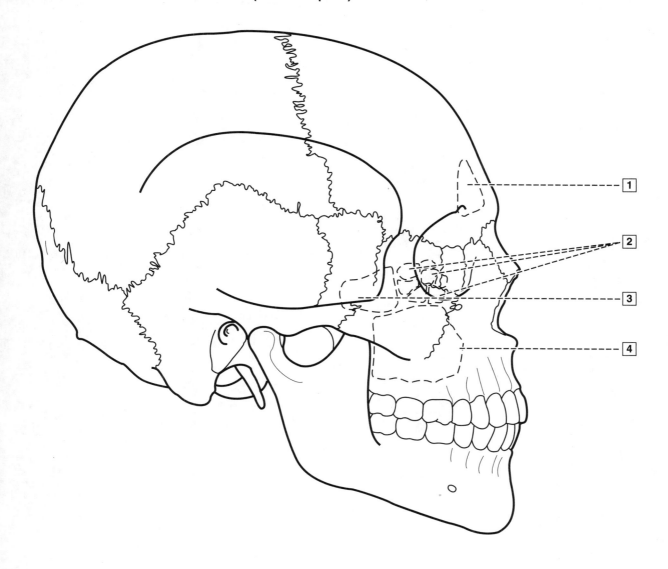

1 Frontal sinus
2 Ethmoidal sinuses
3 Sphenoidal sinus
4 Maxillary sinus

Copyright © 2008 by Saunders, an imprint of Elsevier Inc.

NOTES

Copyright © 2008 by Saunders, an imprint of Elsevier Inc.

FIGURE 4-21 | Temporal fossa and boundaries (lateral view)

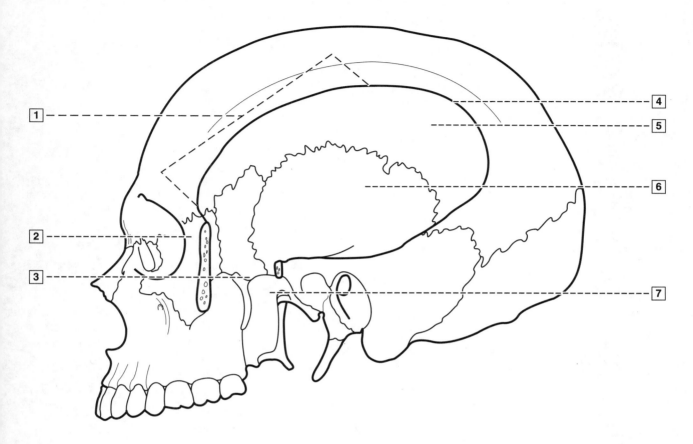

1	Temporal fossa	5	Parietal bone
2	Frontal process of zygomatic bone	6	Squamous portion of temporal bone
3	Infratemporal crest of greater wing of sphenoid bone	7	Infratemporal fossa
4	Inferior temporal line		

NOTES

Copyright © 2008 by Saunders, an imprint of Elsevier Inc.

FIGURE 4-22 | Infratemporal fossa and boundaries (inferior view)

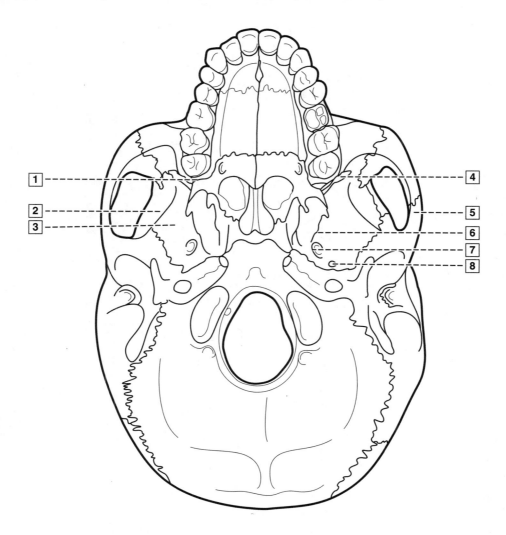

1 Maxillary tuberosity	**5** Zygomatic arch
2 Infratemporal crest of great wing of sphenoid bone	**6** Lateral pterygoid plate of sphenoid bone
3 Infratemporal fossa	**7** Foramen ovale
4 Inferior orbital fissure	**8** Foramen spinosum

Copyright © 2008 by Saunders, an imprint of Elsevier Inc.

NOTES

Copyright © 2008 by Saunders, an imprint of Elsevier Inc.

FIGURE 4-23 | Pterygopalatine fossa and boundaries (oblique lateral view)

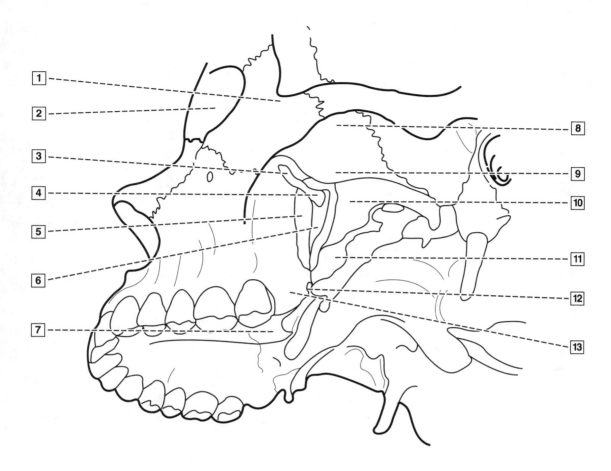

1 Zygomatic arch

2 Orbit

3 Inferior orbital fissure

4 Sphenopalatine foramen

5 Pterygopalatine fossa

6 Pterygomaxillary fissure

7 Palatine bone

8 Temporal fossa

9 Infratemporal crest of the greater wing of sphenoid bone

10 Infratemporal fossa

11 Lateral pterygoid plate of the sphenoid bone

12 Pterygopalatine canal

13 Maxillary tuberosity

Copyright © 2008 by Saunders, an imprint of Elsevier Inc.

NOTES

Copyright © 2008 by Saunders, an imprint of Elsevier Inc.

FIGURE 4-24 | Cervical vertebrae and occipital bone (posterior view)

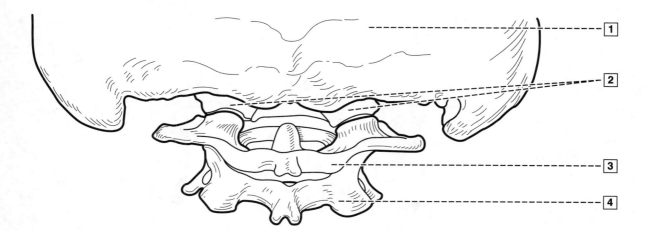

1 Occipital bone

2 Occipital condyle

3 First cervical vertebra, atlas

4 Second cervical vertebra, axis

Copyright © 2008 by Saunders, an imprint of Elsevier Inc.

NOTES

Copyright © 2008 by Saunders, an imprint of Elsevier Inc.

FIGURE 4-25 | First cervical vertebra, atlas (superior view)

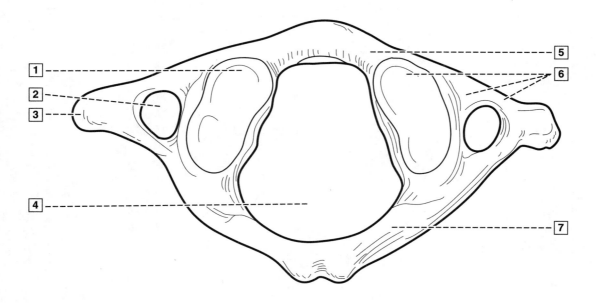

1. Superior articular process
2. Transverse foramen
3. Transverse process
4. Vertebral foramen
5. Anterior arch
6. Lateral mass
7. Posterior arch

Copyright © 2008 by Saunders, an imprint of Elsevier Inc.

NOTES

Copyright © 2008 by Saunders, an imprint of Elsevier Inc.

FIGURE 4-26 ׀ Second cervical vertebra, axis (posterosuperior view)

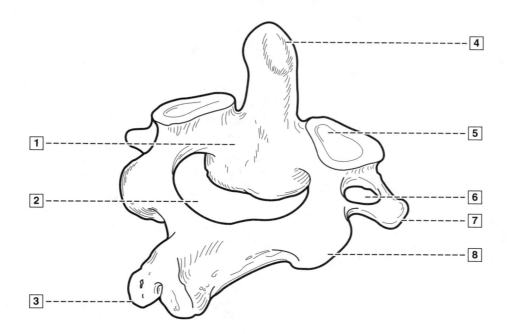

1	Body	**5**	Superior articular process
2	Vertebral foramen	**6**	Transverse foramen
3	Spine	**7**	Transverse process
4	Dens	**8**	Inferior articular process

Copyright © 2008 by Saunders, an imprint of Elsevier Inc.

NOTES

Copyright © 2008 by Saunders, an imprint of Elsevier Inc.

FIGURE 4-27 | Hyoid bone and landmarks (posterolateral view)

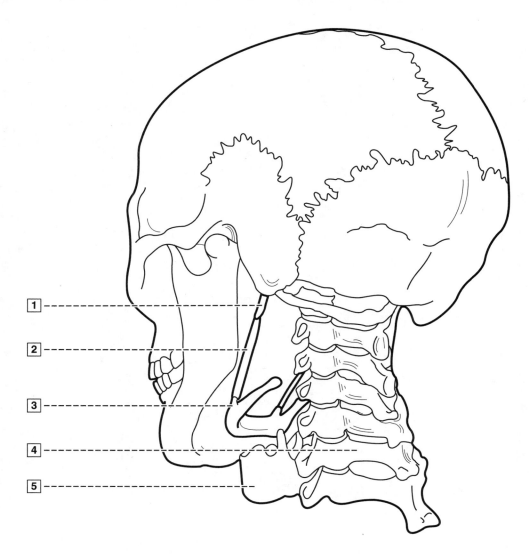

1. Styloid process
2. Styloid muscle
3. Hyoid bone
4. Cervical vertebrae
5. Larynx

Copyright © 2008 by Saunders, an imprint of Elsevier Inc.

NOTES

Copyright © 2008 by Saunders, an imprint of Elsevier Inc.

FIGURE 4-28 | Hyoid bone (anterior view)

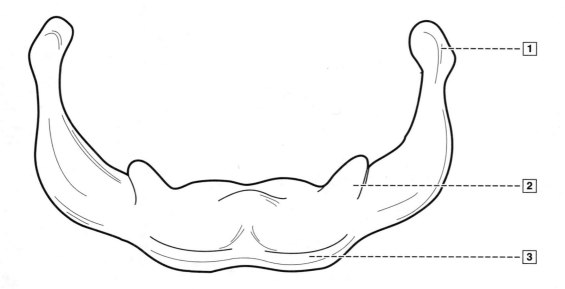

1   Greater cornu
2   Lesser cornu
3   Body

NOTES

Copyright © 2008 by Saunders, an imprint of Elsevier Inc.

FIGURE 5-1 | Sternocleidomastoid muscle (frontal view)

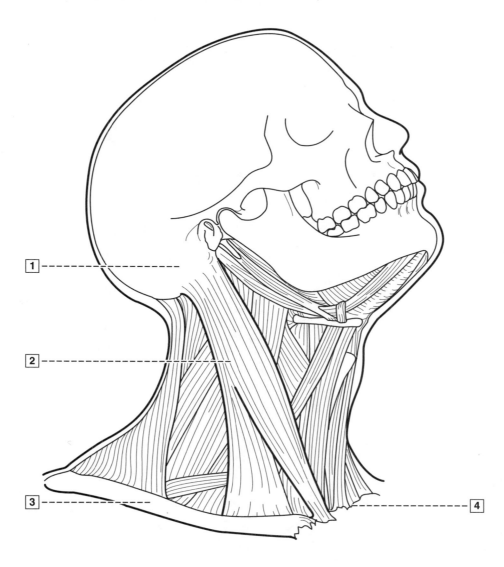

1 Mastoid process of temporal bone
2 Sternocleidomastoid
3 Clavicle
4 Sternum

Copyright © 2008 by Saunders, an imprint of Elsevier Inc.

NOTES

Copyright © 2008 by Saunders, an imprint of Elsevier Inc.

FIGURE 5-2 | Trapezius muscle (posterolateral view)

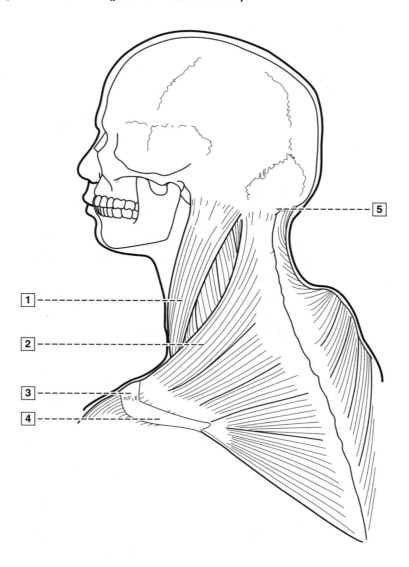

1 Sternocleiodomastoid
2 Trapezius
3 Clavicle
4 Scapula
5 Occipital bone

Copyright © 2008 by Saunders, an imprint of Elsevier Inc.

NOTES

Copyright © 2008 by Saunders, an imprint of Elsevier Inc.

FIGURE 5-3 | Muscles of facial expression (frontal view)

Not all muscles are included in this view.

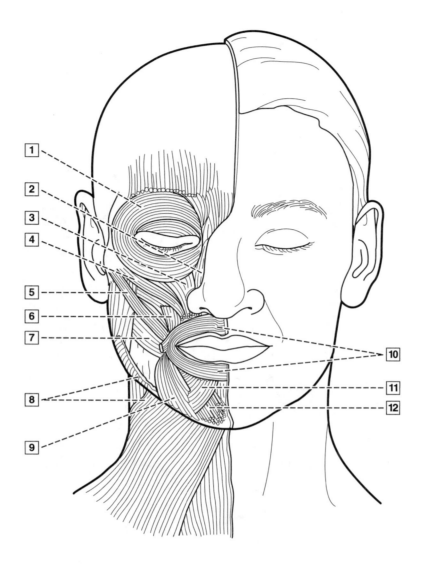

1	Orbicularis oculi	7	Buccinator
2	Levator labii superioris alaeque nasi	8	Platysma
3	Levator labii superioris	9	Depressor anguli oris
4	Zygomaticus minor	10	Orbicularis oris
5	Zygomaticus major	11	Depressor labii inferioris
6	Levator anguli oris	12	Mentalis

Copyright © 2008 by Saunders, an imprint of Elsevier Inc.

NOTES

Copyright © 2008 by Saunders, an imprint of Elsevier Inc.

FIGURE 5-4 | Muscles of facial expression (lateral view)

Not all muscles are included in this view.

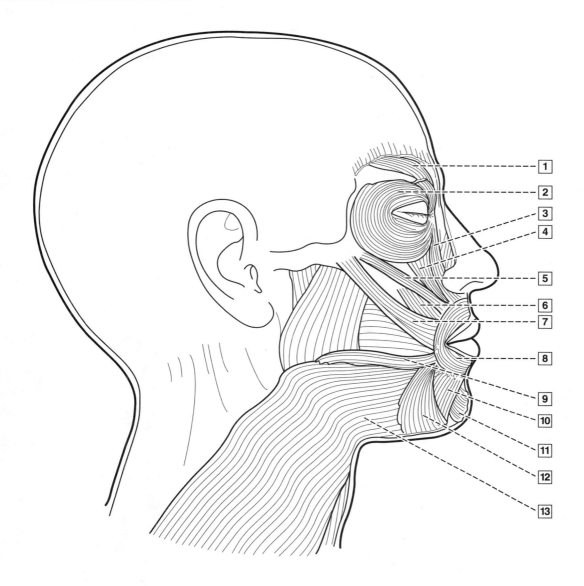

1	Corrugator supercilii	6	Levator anguli oris	11	Mentalis
2	Orbicularis oculi	7	Zygomaticus major	12	Depressor anguli oris
3	Levator labii superioris alaeque nasi	8	Orbicularis oris	13	Platysma
4	Levator labii superioris	9	Risorius		
5	Zygomaticus minor	10	Depressor labii inferioris		

Copyright © 2008 by Saunders, an imprint of Elsevier Inc.

NOTES

Copyright © 2008 by Saunders, an imprint of Elsevier Inc.

FIGURE 5-5 | Muscles of facial expression: epicranial (lateral aspect)

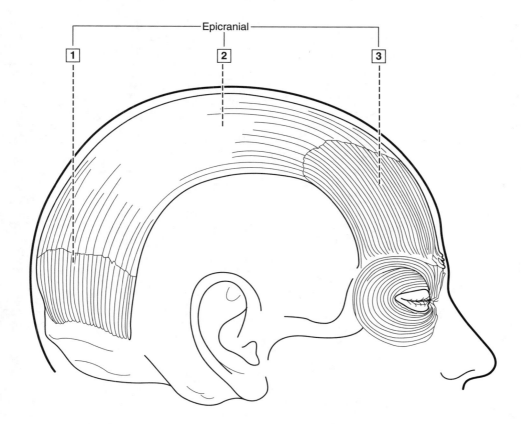

[1] Occipital belly
[2] Epicranial aponeurosis
[3] Frontal belly

NOTES

Copyright © 2008 by Saunders, an imprint of Elsevier Inc.

FIGURE 5-6 | Muscles of facial expression: buccinator (lateral view)

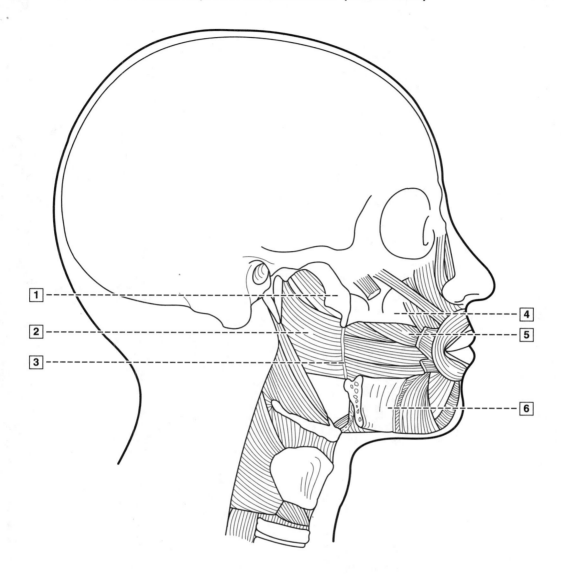

1 Pterygoid plate
2 Superior pharyngeal constrictor
3 Pterygomandibular raphe
4 Maxilla
5 Buccinator
6 Mandible (cut)

Copyright © 2008 by Saunders, an imprint of Elsevier Inc.

NOTES

Copyright © 2008 by Saunders, an imprint of Elsevier Inc.

FIGURE 5-7 | Muscles of mastication: masseter (lateral view)

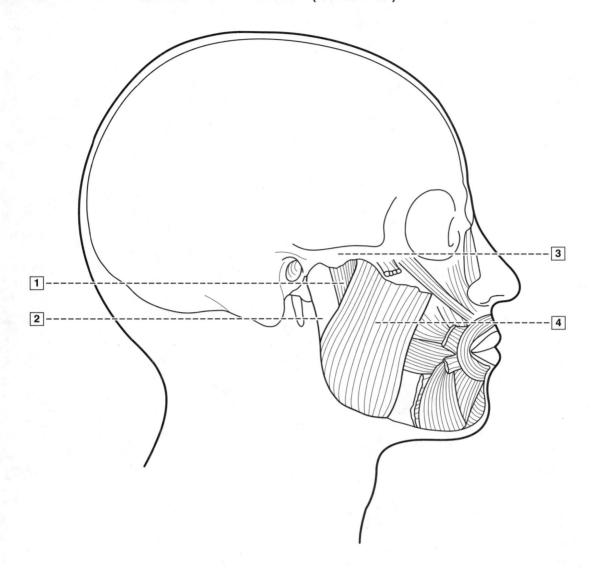

1	Deep head of masseter
2	Ramus of mandible
3	Zygomatic arch
4	Superficial head of masseter

Copyright © 2008 by Saunders, an imprint of Elsevier Inc.

NOTES

Copyright © 2008 by Saunders, an imprint of Elsevier Inc.

FIGURE 5-8 | Muscles of mastication: temporalis (lateral view)

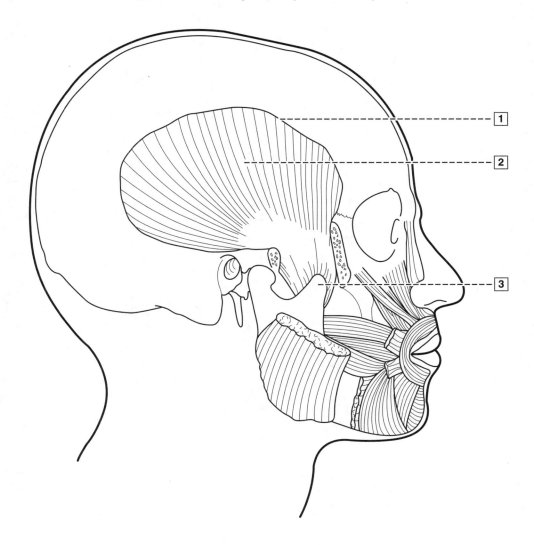

1 Inferior temporal line

2 Temporalis

3 Coronoid process of mandible

Copyright © 2008 by Saunders, an imprint of Elsevier Inc.

NOTES

Copyright © 2008 by Saunders, an imprint of Elsevier Inc.

FIGURE 5-9 | Muscles of mastication: medial and lateral pterygoid (lateral view)

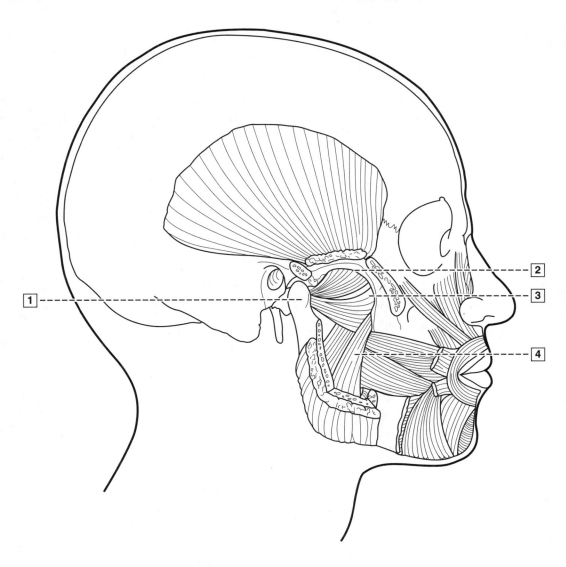

1	Mandibular condyle
2	Superior head of lateral pterygoid
3	Inferior head of lateral pterygoid
4	Medial pterygoid

Copyright © 2008 by Saunders, an imprint of Elsevier Inc.

NOTES

Copyright © 2008 by Saunders, an imprint of Elsevier Inc.

FIGURE 5-10 | Hyoid muscles (anterior view)

Geniohyoid is not included.

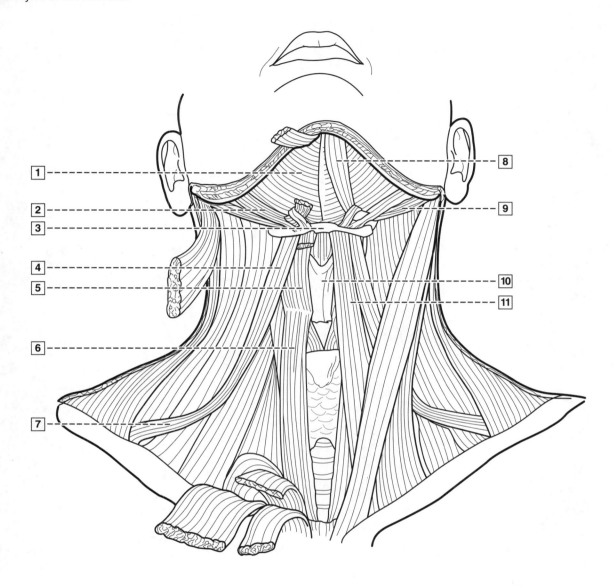

1	Mylohyoid	**7**	Inferior belly of omohyoid
2	Stylohyoid	**8**	Anterior belly of digastric
3	Hyoid bone	**9**	Posterior belly of digastric
4	Superior belly of omohyoid	**10**	Thyroid cartilage
5	Thyrohyoid	**11**	Sternohyoid
6	Sternothyroid		

Copyright © 2008 by Saunders, an imprint of Elsevier Inc.

NOTES

Copyright © 2008 by Saunders, an imprint of Elsevier Inc.

FIGURE 5-11 | Suprahyoid muscles (lateral view)

Geniohyoid is not included.

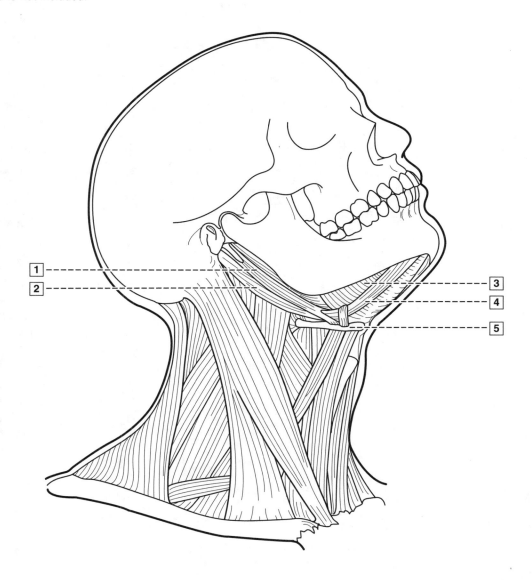

1 Stylohyoid

2 Posterior belly of digastric

3 Mylohyoid

4 Anterior belly of digastric

5 Hyoid bone

Copyright © 2008 by Saunders, an imprint of Elsevier Inc.

NOTES

Copyright © 2008 by Saunders, an imprint of Elsevier Inc.

FIGURE 5-12 | Infrahyoid muscles (lateral view)

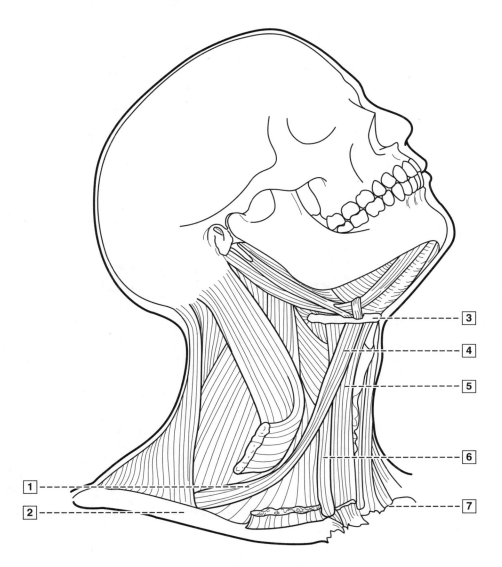

1 Inferior belly of omohyoid
2 Clavicle
3 Hyoid bone
4 Superior belly of omohyoid
5 Sternohyoid
6 Sternothyroid
7 Sternum

NOTES

Copyright © 2008 by Saunders, an imprint of Elsevier Inc.

FIGURE 5-13 │ Suprahyoid muscles: geniohyoid (superior view)

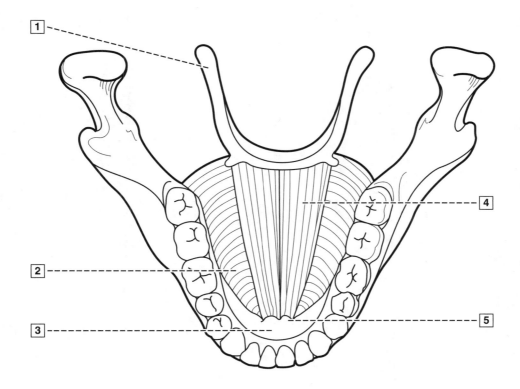

1 Hyoid bone
2 Mylohyoid
3 Mandible
4 Geniohyoid
5 Genial tubercles

Copyright © 2008 by Saunders, an imprint of Elsevier Inc.

NOTES

Copyright © 2008 by Saunders, an imprint of Elsevier Inc.

FIGURE 5-14 | Tongue muscles (superior view)

The palatoglossus muscle of the soft palate is shown.

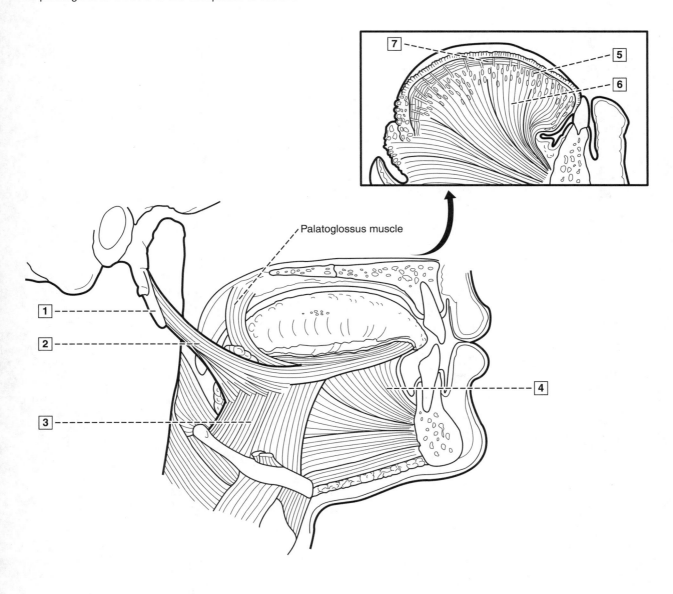

Palatoglossus muscle

Extrinsic

1 Styloid process

2 Styloglossus

3 Hyoglossus

4 Genioglossus

Intrinsic

5 Transverse

6 Vertical

7 Longitudinal

NOTES

Copyright © 2008 by Saunders, an imprint of Elsevier Inc.

FIGURE 5-15 | Muscles of the pharynx (posterior view)

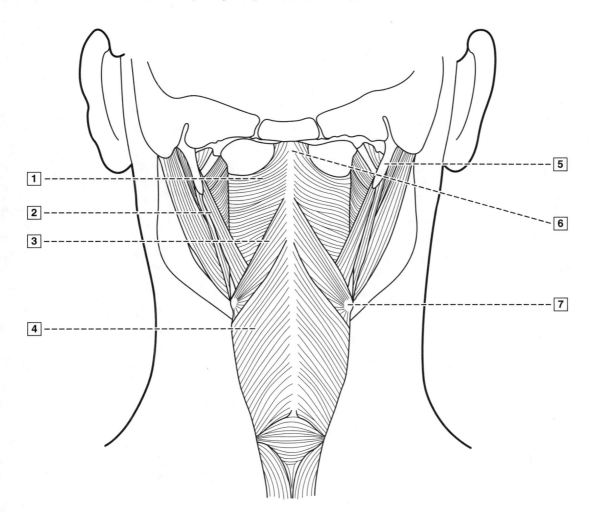

1	Superior pharyngeal constrictor
2	Stylopharyngeus
3	Middle pharyngeal constrictor
4	Inferior pharyngeal constrictor
5	Styloid process
6	Median pharyngeal raphe
7	Hyoid bone

Copyright © 2008 by Saunders, an imprint of Elsevier Inc.

NOTES

Copyright © 2008 by Saunders, an imprint of Elsevier Inc.

FIGURE 5-16 │ Muscles of the pharynx (lateral view)

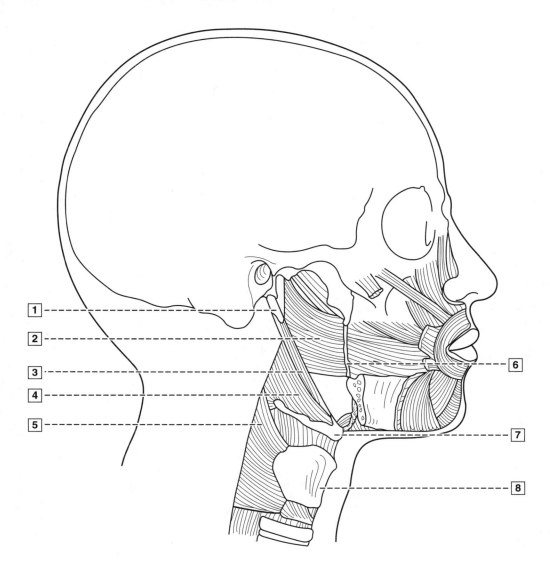

1	Styloid process
2	Superior pharyngeal constrictor
3	Stylopharyngeus
4	Middle pharyngeal constrictor
5	Inferior pharyngeal constrictor
6	Pterygomandibular raphe
7	Hyoid bone
8	Thyroid cartilage

Copyright © 2008 by Saunders, an imprint of Elsevier Inc.

NOTES

Copyright © 2008 by Saunders, an imprint of Elsevier Inc.

FIGURE 5-17 | Muscles of the soft palate (posterior and cutaway views)

The palatoglossus muscle is shown with the muscles of the tongue.

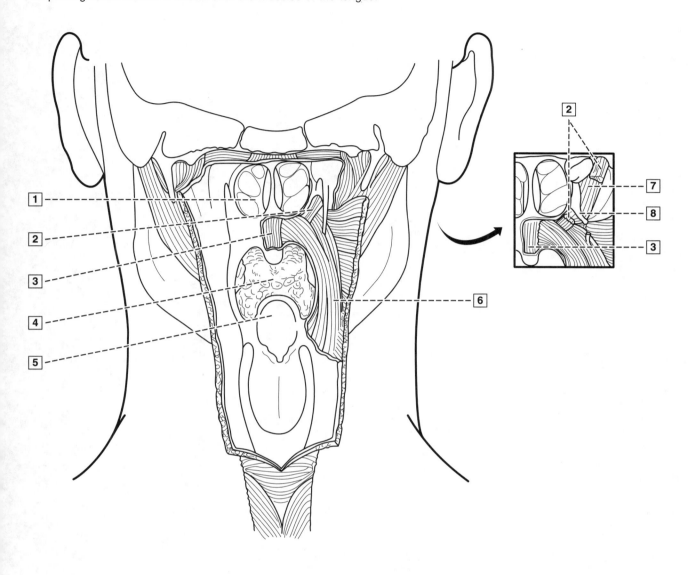

1	Nasal cavity	**5**	Epiglottis
2	Levator veli palatini	**6**	Palatopharyngeus
3	Muscle of uvula	**7**	Tensor veli palatini
4	Dorsal surface of tongue	**8**	Hamulus

Copyright © 2008 by Saunders, an imprint of Elsevier Inc.

NOTES

Copyright © 2008 by Saunders, an imprint of Elsevier Inc.

FIGURE 6-1 | Pathways to and from the heart—arteries and veins (frontal view)

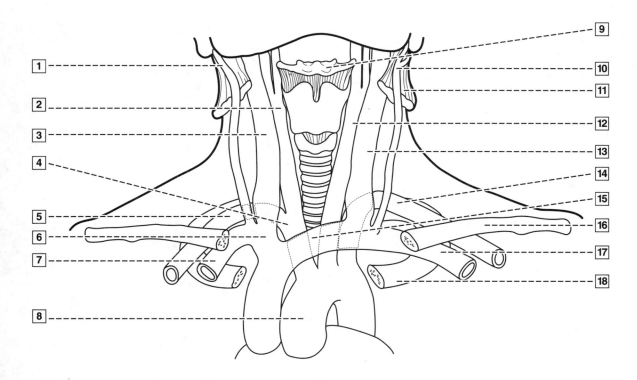

1	Right external jugular vein	10	Left external jugular vein
2	Right common carotid artery	11	Sternocleidomastoid muscle (cut)
3	Right internal jugular vein	12	Left common carotid artery
4	Brachiocephalic artery	13	Left internal jugular vein
5	Right subclavian artery	14	Left subclavian artery
6	Right brachiocephalic vein	15	Left brachiocephalic vein
7	Right subclavian vein	16	Clavicle (cut)
8	Aorta	17	Left subclavian vein
9	Hyoid bone	18	First rib (cut)

NOTES

Copyright © 2008 by Saunders, an imprint of Elsevier Inc.

FIGURE 6-2 | Common carotid artery: internal and external arteries (lateral view)

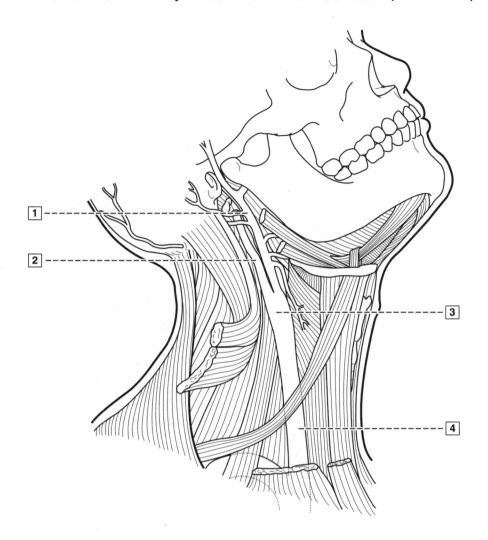

1	External carotid
2	Internal carotid
3	Carotid sinus
4	Common carotid

Copyright © 2008 by Saunders, an imprint of Elsevier Inc.

NOTES

Copyright © 2008 by Saunders, an imprint of Elsevier Inc.

FIGURE 6-3 | Common carotid artery: external carotid (lateral view)

The medial branch, the ascending pharyngeal, is not shown.

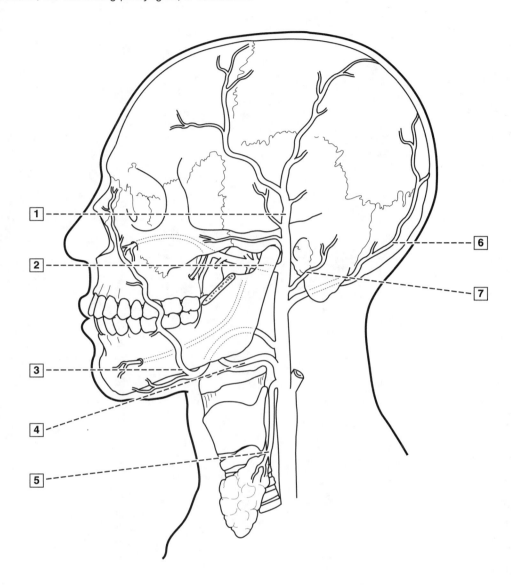

Terminal branches

1. Maxillary
2. Superficial temporal

Anterior branches

3. Facial
4. Lingual
5. Superior thyroid

Posterior branches

6. Occipital
7. Posterior auricular

Copyright © 2008 by Saunders, an imprint of Elsevier Inc.

NOTES

Copyright © 2008 by Saunders, an imprint of Elsevier Inc.

FIGURE 6-4 | External carotid artery: maxillary (lateral view)

Greater and lesser palatine arteries are not shown.

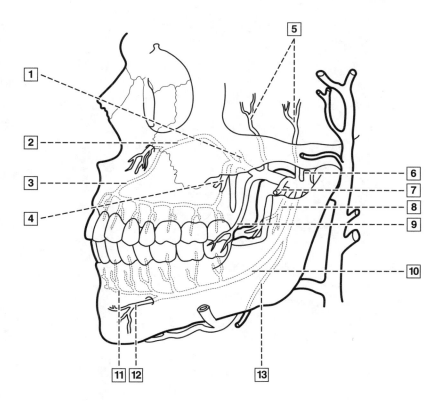

1	Sphenopalatine (cut)	8	Pterygoids
2	Infraorbital	9	Buccal
3	Anterior superior alveolar (branch of infraorbital)	10	Inferior alveolar
4	Posterior superior alveolar (portion cut)	11	Incisive
5	Deep temporals	12	Mental
6	Middle meningeal (cut)	13	Mylohyoid
7	Masseteric (cut)		

11 Incisive ⎫
12 Mental ⎬ Branches of inferior alveolar
13 Mylohyoid ⎭

Copyright © 2008 by Saunders, an imprint of Elsevier Inc.

NOTES

Copyright © 2008 by Saunders, an imprint of Elsevier Inc.

FIGURE 6-5 | Maxillary artery: palatal branches (sagittal section of nasal cavity)

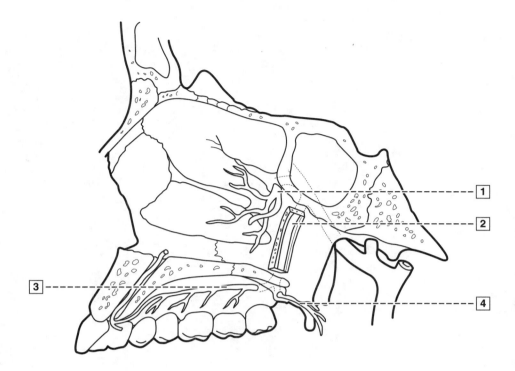

1 Sphenopalatine

2 Descending palatine

3 Greater palatine

4 Lesser palatine

Copyright © 2008 by Saunders, an imprint of Elsevier Inc.

NOTES

Copyright © 2008 by Saunders, an imprint of Elsevier Inc.

FIGURE 6-6 | External carotid artery: superficial temporal (lateral view)

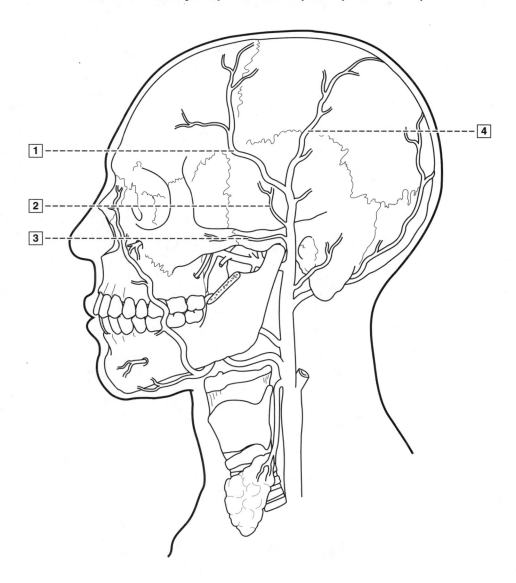

1 Frontal branch
2 Middle temporal
3 Transverse facial
4 Parietal branch

Copyright © 2008 by Saunders, an imprint of Elsevier Inc.

NOTES

Copyright © 2008 by Saunders, an imprint of Elsevier Inc.

FIGURE 6-7 | External carotid artery: anterior branches (sagittal section)

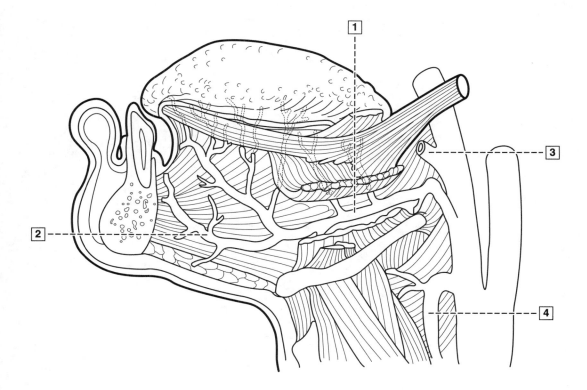

1 Lingual
2 Sublingual
3 Facial (cut)
4 Superior thyroid

Copyright © 2008 by Saunders, an imprint of Elsevier Inc.

NOTES

Copyright © 2008 by Saunders, an imprint of Elsevier Inc.

FIGURE 6-8 | External carotid artery: facial (lateral view)

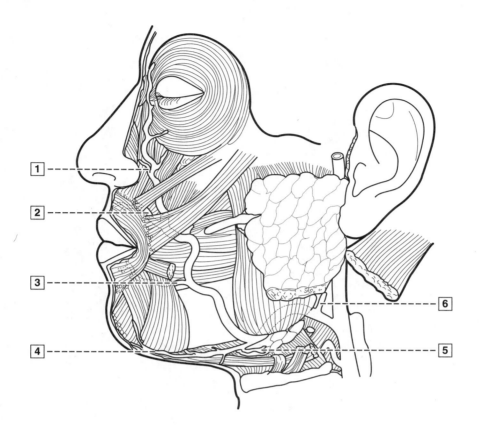

1 Angular

2 Superior labial

3 Inferior labial

4 Submental

5 Glandular branches

6 Ascending palatine

Copyright © 2008 by Saunders, an imprint of Elsevier Inc.

NOTES

Copyright © 2008 by Saunders, an imprint of Elsevier Inc.

FIGURE 6-9 | External carotid artery: posterior branches (lateral view)

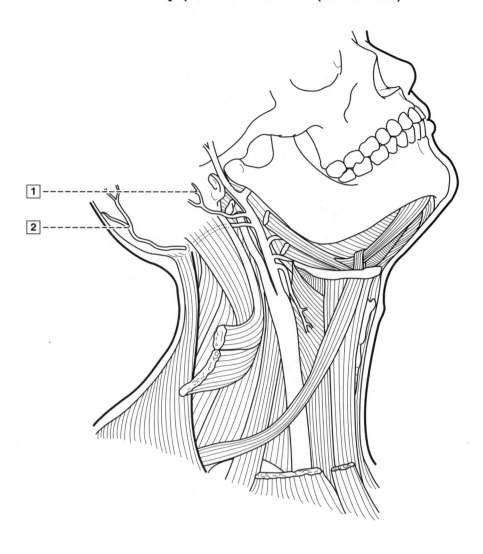

1 Posterior auricular
2 Occipital

NOTES

 Copyright © 2008 by Saunders, an imprint of Elsevier Inc.

FIGURE 6-10 | Vascular system: internal jugular and facial veins *plus* vessel anastomoses (lateral view)

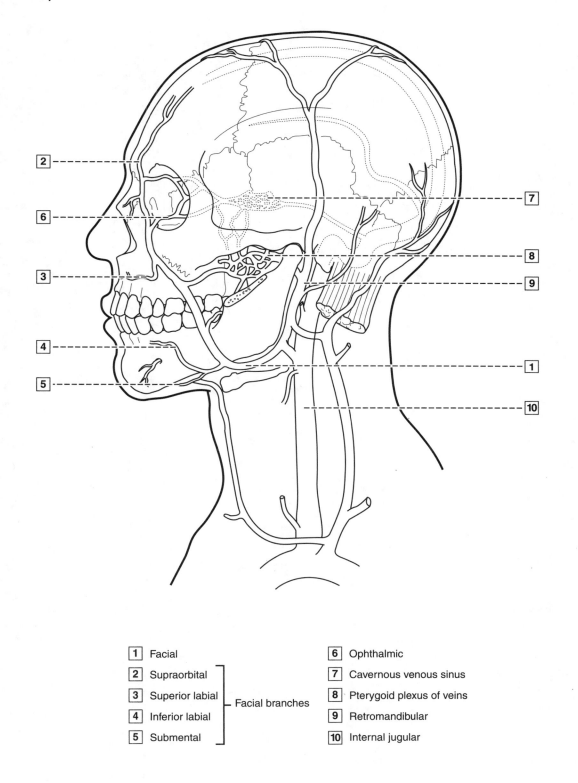

1 Facial	6 Ophthalmic
2 Supraorbital	7 Cavernous venous sinus
3 Superior labial	8 Pterygoid plexus of veins
4 Inferior labial	9 Retromandibular
5 Submental	10 Internal jugular

2, 3, 4, 5 — Facial branches

Copyright © 2008 by Saunders, an imprint of Elsevier Inc.

NOTES

Copyright © 2008 by Saunders, an imprint of Elsevier Inc.

FIGURE 6-11 | Vascular system: external jugular and retromandibular veins *plus* vessel anastomoses (lateral view)

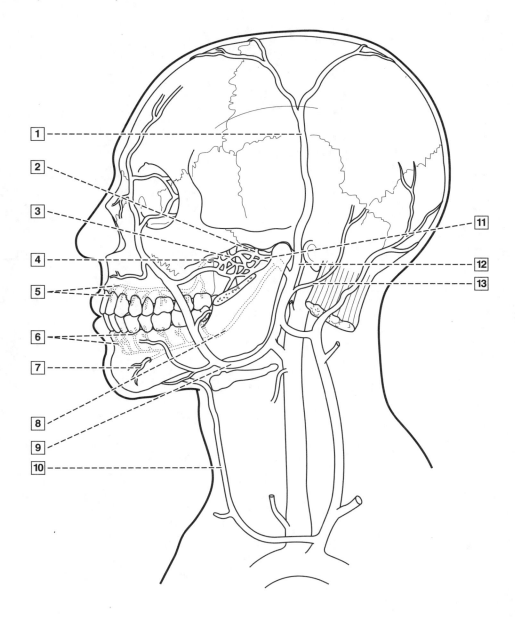

1 Superficial temporal		**7** Mental branch of inferior alveolar	
2 Middle meningeal		**8** Inferior alveolar	
3 Pterygoid plexus of veins		**9** Facial	
4 Posterior superior alveolar		**10** Anterior jugular	
5 Alveolar and dental branches of posterior superior alveolar		**11** Maxillary	
6 Alveolar and dental branches of inferior alveolar		**12** Retromandibular	
		13 Posterior auricular	

Copyright © 2008 by Saunders, an imprint of Elsevier Inc.

NOTES

Copyright © 2008 by Saunders, an imprint of Elsevier Inc.

FIGURE 7-1 | Lacrimal apparatus (frontal and cutaway views)

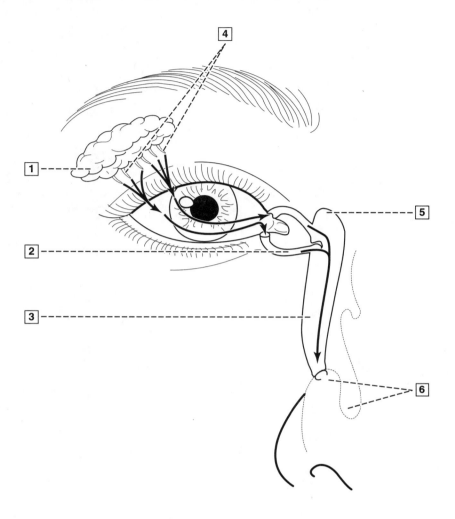

1 Lacrimal gland
2 Lacrimal canal
3 Nasolacrimal duct
4 Lacrimal ducts
5 Lacrimal sac
6 Inferior meatus and turbinate

Copyright © 2008 by Saunders, an imprint of Elsevier Inc.

NOTES

Copyright © 2008 by Saunders, an imprint of Elsevier Inc.

FIGURE 7-2 ǀ Major salivary glands and ducts (ventral and frontal aspects with internal views)

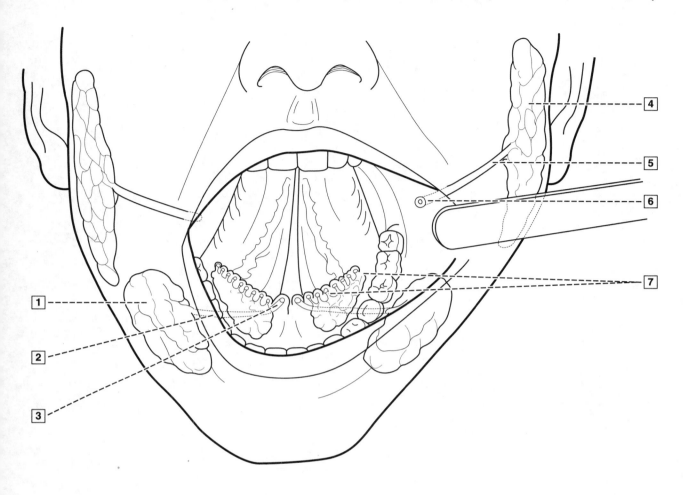

1 Submandibular gland
2 Submandibular duct
3 Sublingual caruncle
4 Parotid gland
5 Parotid duct
6 Parotid papilla
7 Sublingual ducts

Copyright © 2008 by Saunders, an imprint of Elsevier Inc.

NOTES

Copyright © 2008 by Saunders, an imprint of Elsevier Inc.

FIGURE 7-3 | Salivary glands: acini and ducts (microscopic view)

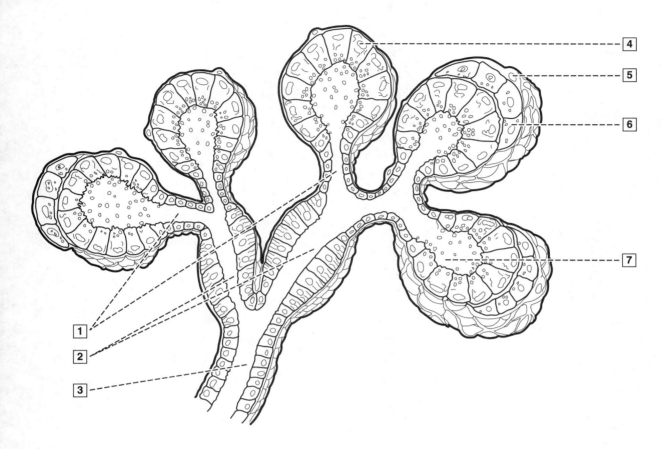

1	Intercalated ducts	5	Myoepithelial cell
2	Striated ducts	6	Serous demilune
3	Excretory duct	7	Lumen of acinus
4	Mucous cell		

Copyright © 2008 by Saunders, an imprint of Elsevier Inc.

NOTES

Copyright © 2008 by Saunders, an imprint of Elsevier Inc.

FIGURE 7-4 | Major salivary glands: parotid gland (lateral view)

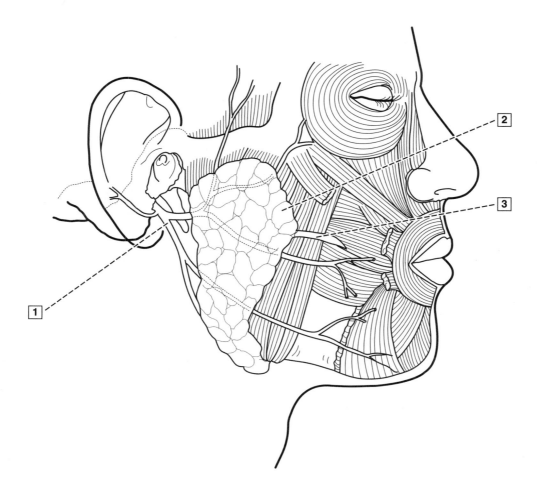

1 Facial nerve (VII)
2 Parotid gland
3 Parotid duct

Copyright © 2008 by Saunders, an imprint of Elsevier Inc.

NOTES

Copyright © 2008 by Saunders, an imprint of Elsevier Inc.

FIGURE 7-5 | Major salivary glands: submandibular gland (lateral view)

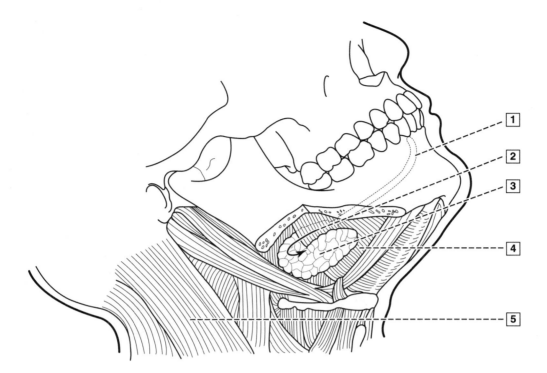

1 Submandibular duct

2 Deep lobe, submandibular gland

3 Superficial lobe, submandibular gland

4 Mylohyoid muscle

5 Sternocleidomastoid muscle

Copyright © 2008 by Saunders, an imprint of Elsevier Inc.

NOTES

Copyright © 2008 by Saunders, an imprint of Elsevier Inc.

FIGURE 7-6 ┃ Major salivary glands: sublingual gland (ventral and frontal aspects with internal views)

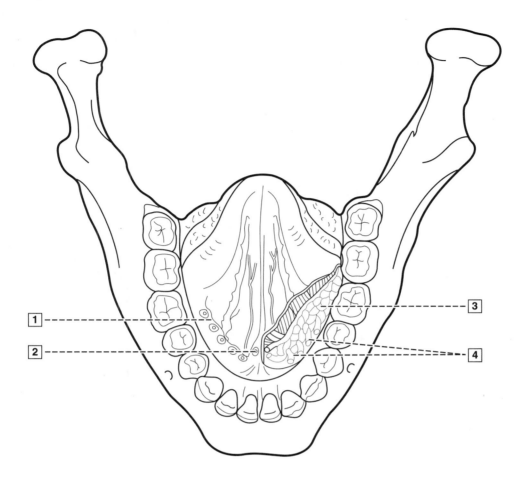

1 Sublingual fold
2 Sublingual caruncle
3 Sublingual gland
4 Sublingual ducts

Copyright © 2008 by Saunders, an imprint of Elsevier Inc.

NOTES

Copyright © 2008 by Saunders, an imprint of Elsevier Inc.

FIGURE 7-7 | Glandular tissue: thyroid and parathyroid glands (anterior and posterior views)

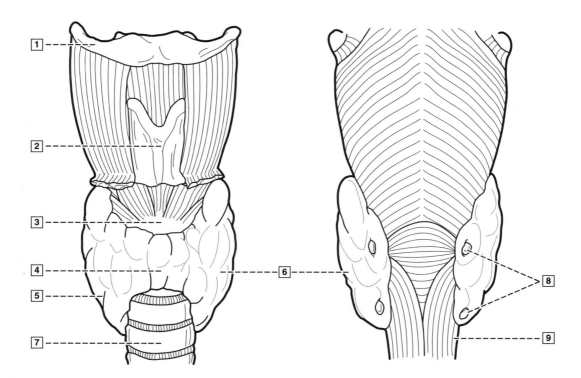

1 Hyoid bone
2 Thyroid cartilage
3 Cricoid cartilage
4 Isthmus
5 Right lobe of thyroid gland
6 Left lobe of thyroid gland
7 Trachea
8 Parathyroid glands
9 Esophagus

Copyright © 2008 by Saunders, an imprint of Elsevier Inc.

NOTES

Copyright © 2008 by Saunders, an imprint of Elsevier Inc.

FIGURE 7-8 | Glandular tissue: thymus (anterior view)

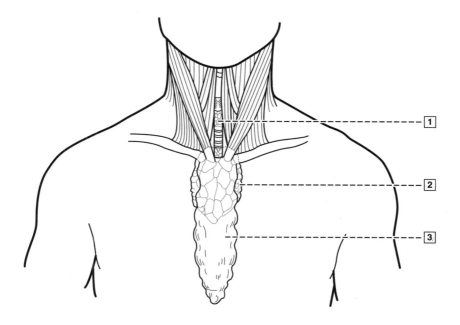

1	Thyroid gland
2	Thymus
3	Sternum

NOTES

Copyright © 2008 by Saunders, an imprint of Elsevier Inc.

FIGURE 8-1 | Brain (ventral view)

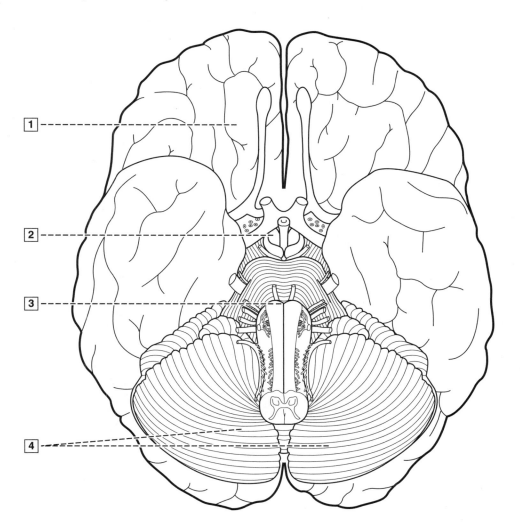

1 Cerebral hemisphere
2 Diencephalon
3 Brainstem
4 Cerebellum

Copyright © 2008 by Saunders, an imprint of Elsevier Inc.

NOTES

Copyright © 2008 by Saunders, an imprint of Elsevier Inc.

FIGURE 8-2 | Brain and spinal cord (lateral sagittal view)

The brain and spinal cord together form the central nervous system.

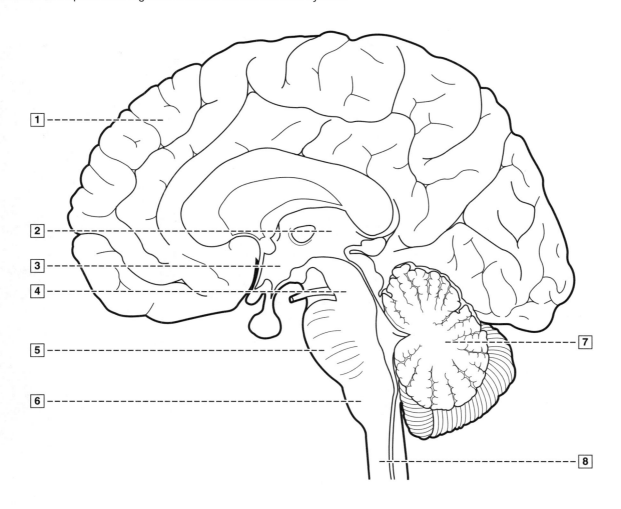

1	Cerebral hemisphere	**7**	Cerebellum
Diencephalon		**8**	Spinal cord
2	Thalamus		
3	Hypothalamus		
Brainstem			
4	Midbrain		
5	Pons		
6	Medulla		

NOTES

Copyright © 2008 by Saunders, an imprint of Elsevier Inc.

FIGURE 8-3 | Brain and cranial nerves (ventral surface showing nerve attachment)

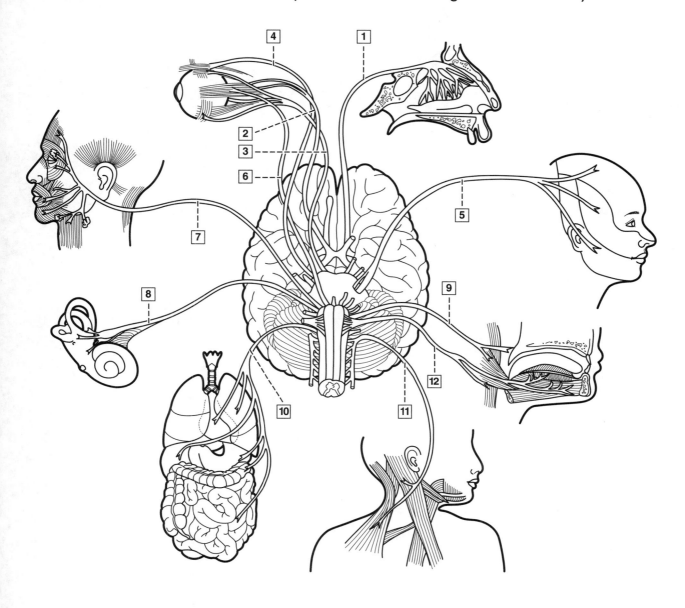

1	Olfactory nerve (I)	**7**	Facial nerve (VII)
2	Optic nerve (II)	**8**	Vestibulocochlear nerve (VIII)
3	Oculomotor nerve (III)	**9**	Glossopharyngeal nerve (IX)
4	Trochlear nerve (IV)	**10**	Vagus nerve (X)
5	Trigeminal nerve (V)	**11**	Accessory nerve (XI)
6	Abducens nerve (VI)	**12**	Hypoglossal nerve (XII)

Copyright © 2008 by Saunders, an imprint of Elsevier Inc.

NOTES

Copyright © 2008 by Saunders, an imprint of Elsevier Inc.

FIGURE 8-4 | Cranial nerves and skull (internal view of the skull base)

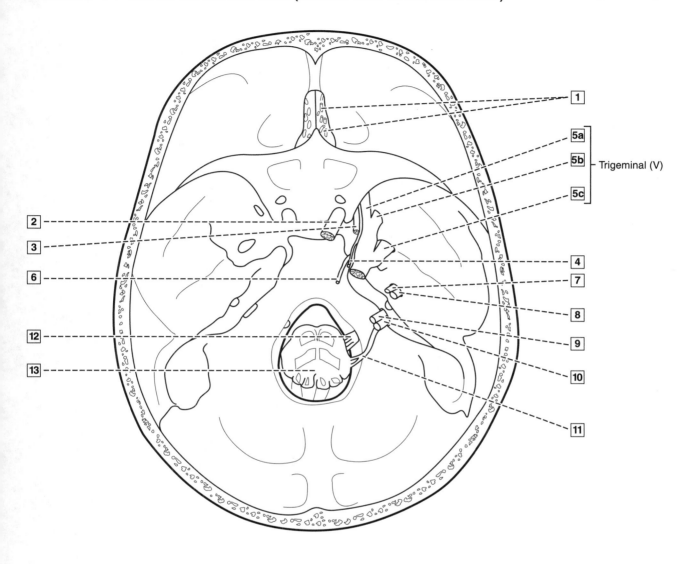

1	Olfactory nerve (I)	6	Abducent nerve (VI)
2	Optic nerve (II)	7	Facial nerve (VII)
3	Oculomotor nerve (III)	8	Vestibulocochlear nerve (VIII)
4	Trochlear nerve (IV)	9	Glossopharyngeal nerve (IX)
Trigeminal nerve (V)		10	Vagus nerve (X)
5a	Ophthalmic nerve	11	Accessory nerve (XI)
5b	Maxillary nerve	12	Hypoglossal nerve (XII)
5c	Mandibular nerve	13	Spinal cord

Copyright © 2008 by Saunders, an imprint of Elsevier Inc.

NOTES

Copyright © 2008 by Saunders, an imprint of Elsevier Inc.

FIGURE 8-5 | Cranial nerve supply to the oral cavity

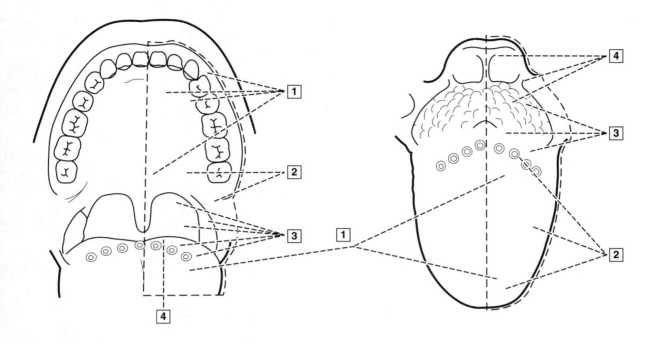

1	Trigeminal nerve (V)
2	Facial nerve (VII)
3	Glossopharyngeal nerve (IX)
4	Vagus nerve (X)

NOTES

Copyright © 2008 by Saunders, an imprint of Elsevier Inc.

FIGURE 8-6 │ Trigeminal nerve (V): ganglion and divisions (lateral view)

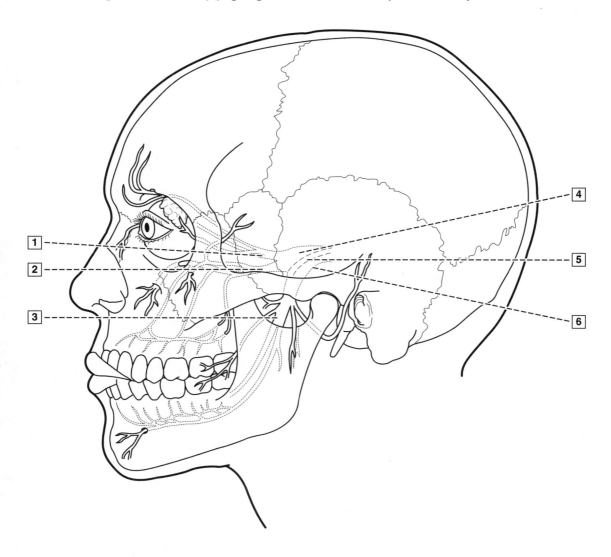

1 Ophthalmic (V₁)

2 Maxillary (V₂)

3 Mandibular (V₃)

4 Trigeminal ganglion

5 Motor root

6 Sensory root

Copyright © 2008 by Saunders, an imprint of Elsevier Inc.

NOTES

Copyright © 2008 by Saunders, an imprint of Elsevier Inc.

FIGURE 8-7 | Trigeminal nerve (V): ophthalmic (V₁) (lateral cutaway view)

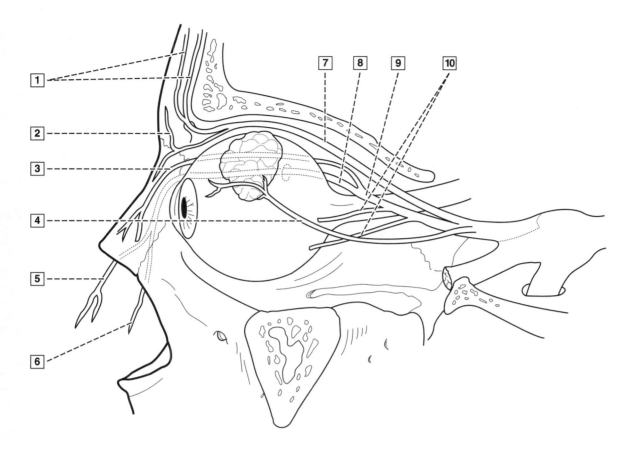

1	Supraorbital	**6**	Internal nasal
2	Supratrochlear	**7**	Frontal
3	Infratrochlear	**8**	Anterior ethmoidal
4	Lacrimal	**9**	Nasociliary
5	External nasal	**10**	Ciliary

Copyright © 2008 by Saunders, an imprint of Elsevier Inc.

NOTES

Copyright © 2008 by Saunders, an imprint of Elsevier Inc.

FIGURE 8-8 | Trigeminal nerve (V): maxillary (V₂) (lateral view)

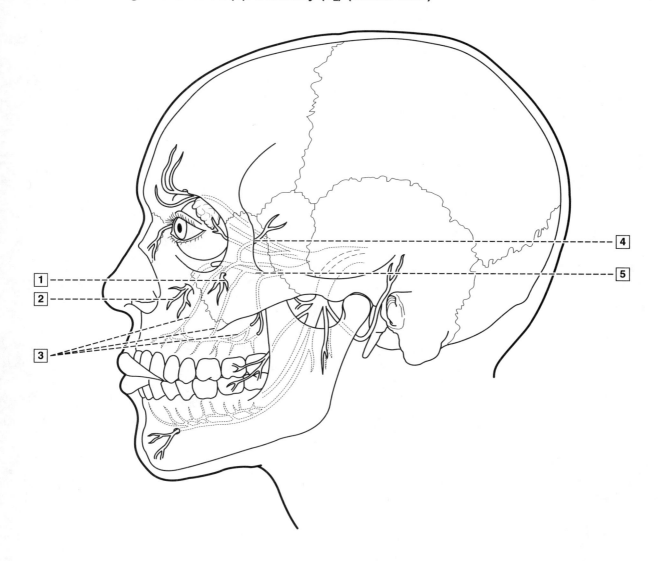

1 Zygomaticofacial
2 Infraorbital
3 Superior alveolars
4 Zygomaticotemporal
5 Zygomatic

Copyright © 2008 by Saunders, an imprint of Elsevier Inc.

NOTES

Copyright © 2008 by Saunders, an imprint of Elsevier Inc.

FIGURE 8-9 | Maxillary nerve (V₂): major branches (lateral view)

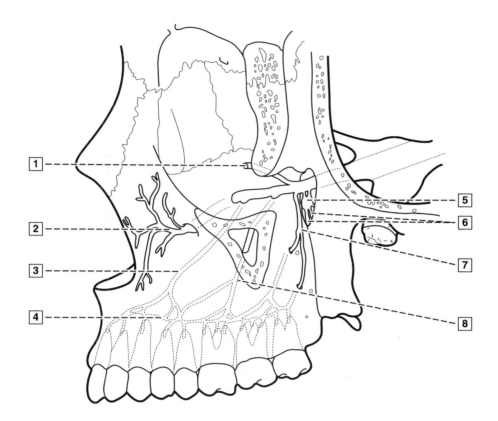

1	Zygomatic	5	Pterygopalatine ganglion
2	Infraorbital	6	Greater and lesser palatine
3	Anterior superior alveolar	7	Posterior superior alveolar
4	Dental plexus	8	Middle superior alveolar

NOTES

Copyright © 2008 by Saunders, an imprint of Elsevier Inc.

FIGURE 8-10 | Maxillary nerve (V₂): palatine branches (medial view of the nasal wall)

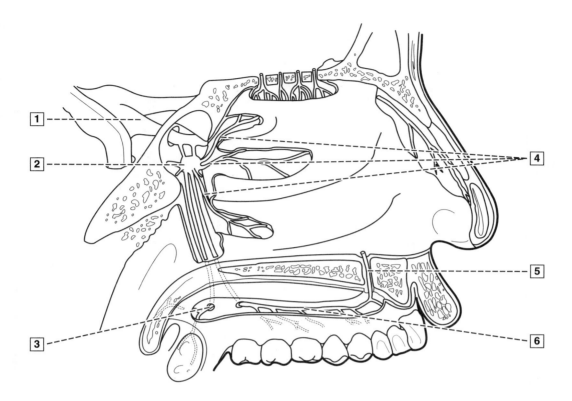

1	Maxillary (V₂)	**4**	Lateral nasal branches
2	Pterygopalatine ganglion	**5**	Nasopalatine (cut)
3	Lesser palatine	**6**	Greater palatine

Copyright © 2008 by Saunders, an imprint of Elsevier Inc.

NOTES

Copyright © 2008 by Saunders, an imprint of Elsevier Inc.

FIGURE 8-11 | Trigeminal nerve (V): mandibular (V₃) (lateral view)

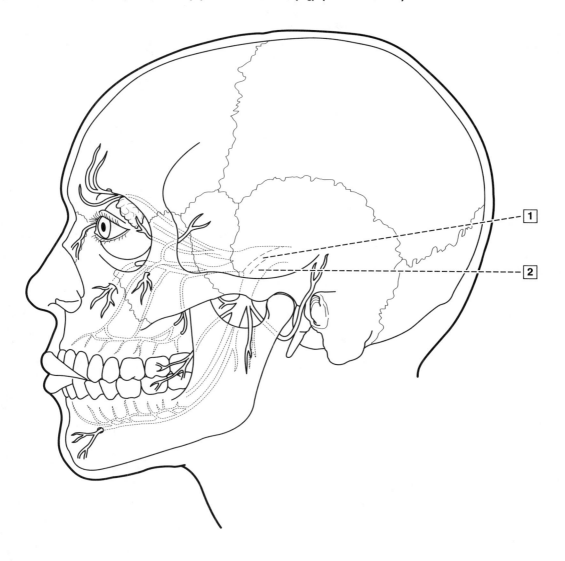

| 1 | Motor root |
| 2 | Sensory root |

NOTES

Copyright © 2008 by Saunders, an imprint of Elsevier Inc.

FIGURE 8-12 | Mandibular nerve (V₃): anterior trunk (lateral view)

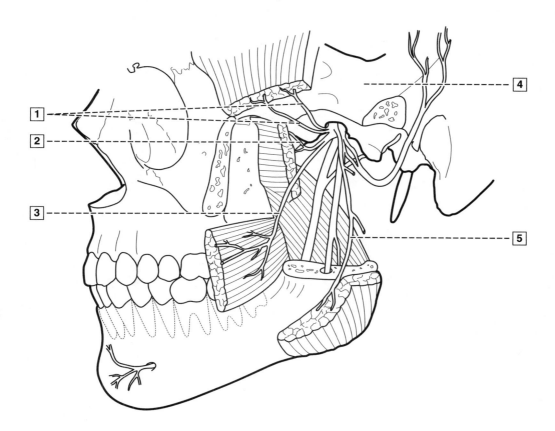

1. Anterior and posterior deep temporal
2. Lateral pterygoid
3. Buccal
4. Trigeminal ganglion location
5. Masseteric

Copyright © 2008 by Saunders, an imprint of Elsevier Inc.

NOTES

Copyright © 2008 by Saunders, an imprint of Elsevier Inc.

FIGURE 8-13 | Mandibular nerve (V₃): posterior trunk (lateral view)

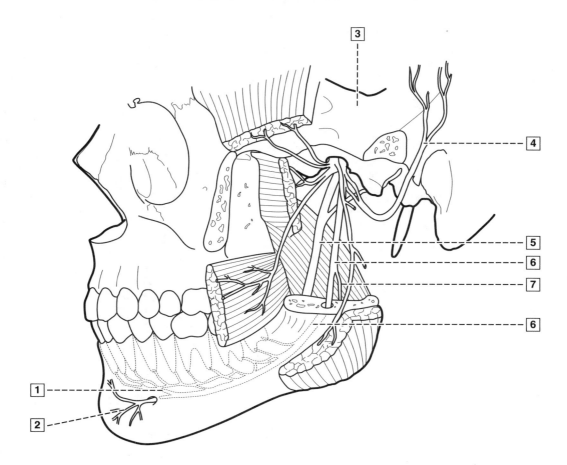

1	Incisive	**5**	Lingual
2	Mental	**6**	Inferior alveolar
3	Location of trigeminal ganglion	**7**	Mylohyoid
4	Auriculotemporal		

Copyright © 2008 by Saunders, an imprint of Elsevier Inc.

NOTES

Copyright © 2008 by Saunders, an imprint of Elsevier Inc.

FIGURE 8-14 | Mandibular nerve (V₃): motor and sensory branches (medial view)

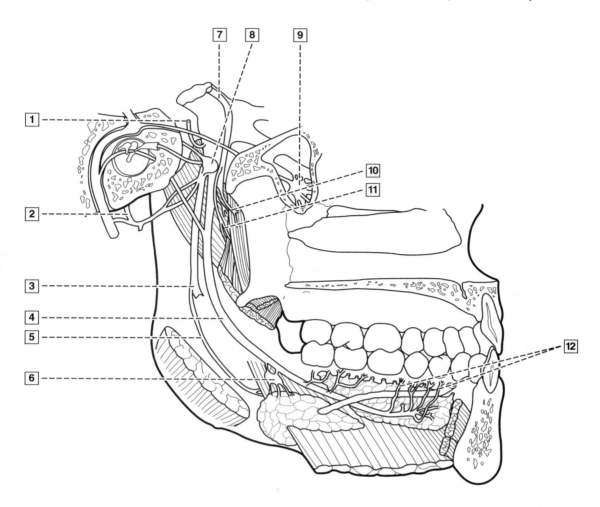

1	Middle meningeal		7	Motor root of trigeminal nerve
2	Auriculotemporal		8	Otic ganglion
3	Inferior alveolar		9	Pterygopalatine ganglion
4	Lingual		10	Nerve to tensor veli palatini muscle
5	Mylohyoid		11	Nerve to medial pterygoid muscle
6	Submandibular ganglion		12	Branches to tongue

Copyright © 2008 by Saunders, an imprint of Elsevier Inc.

NOTES

Copyright © 2008 by Saunders, an imprint of Elsevier Inc.

FIGURE 8-15 | Facial (VII) and trigeminal (V) nerves (medial view)

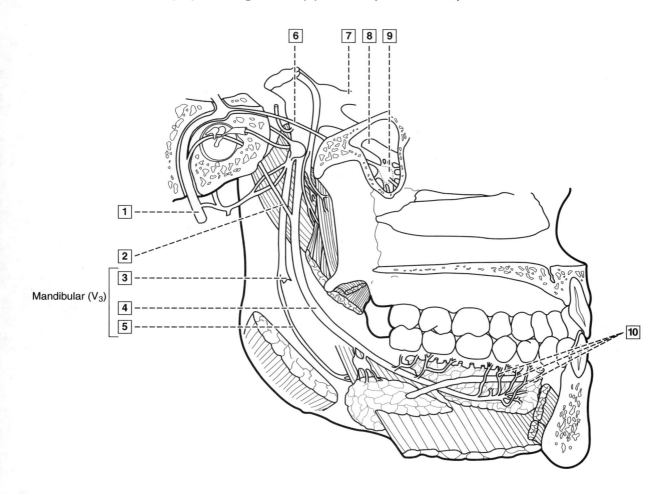

1	Facial (VII)	6	Greater petrosal
2	Chorda tympani	7	Ophthalmic (V_1)
3	Inferior alveolar	8	Maxillary (V_2)
4	Lingual	9	Pterygopalatine ganglion
5	Mylohyoid	10	Sensory fibers from tongue

Copyright © 2008 by Saunders, an imprint of Elsevier Inc.

NOTES

Copyright © 2008 by Saunders, an imprint of Elsevier Inc.

FIGURE 8-16 | Facial nerve (VII) (lateral view)

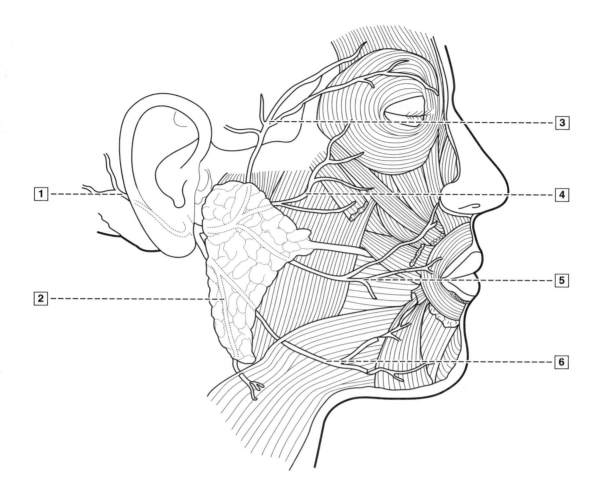

1 Posterior auricular
2 Cervical branch
3 Temporal branches
4 Zygomatic branches
5 Buccal branches
6 Mandibular branch

NOTES

Copyright © 2008 by Saunders, an imprint of Elsevier Inc.

FIGURE 9-1 | Upper body lymphatics (frontal view)

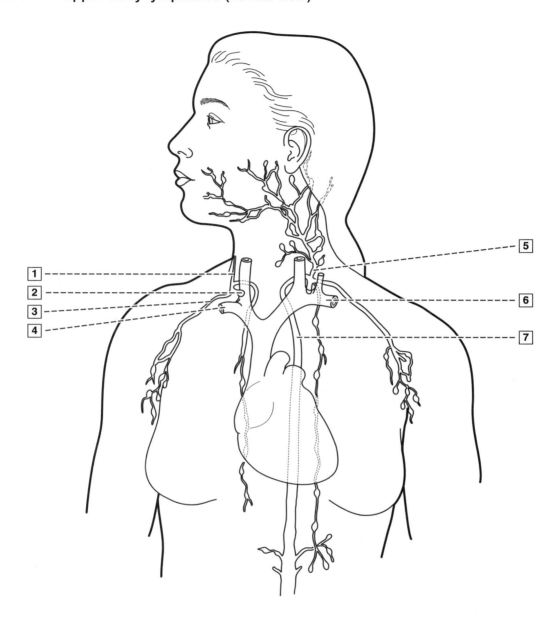

Right side

1 Right jugular trunk

2 Right lymphatic duct

3 Right subclavian trunk

4 Right subclavian vein

Left side

5 Left jugular trunk

6 Left subclavian trunk

7 Thoracic duct

Copyright © 2008 by Saunders, an imprint of Elsevier Inc.

NOTES

Copyright © 2008 by Saunders, an imprint of Elsevier Inc.

FIGURE 9-2 | Superficial nodes of the head (lateral view)

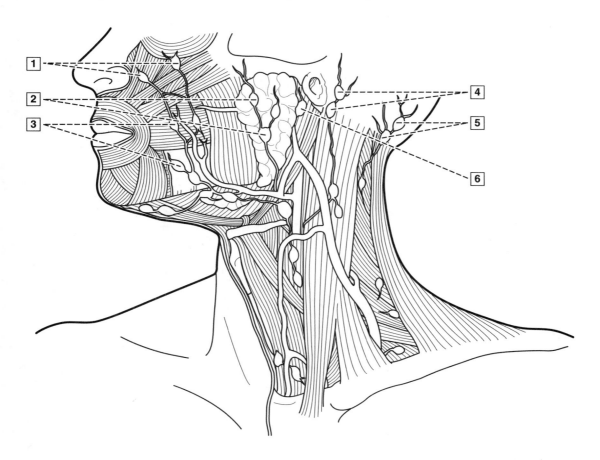

1	Facial nodes
2	Superficial parotid nodes
3	Facial nodes
4	Retroauricular nodes
5	Occipital nodes
6	Anterior auricular node

Copyright © 2008 by Saunders, an imprint of Elsevier Inc.

NOTES

Copyright © 2008 by Saunders, an imprint of Elsevier Inc.

FIGURE 9-3 | Deep nodes of the head (lateral view)

The parotid gland is outlined.

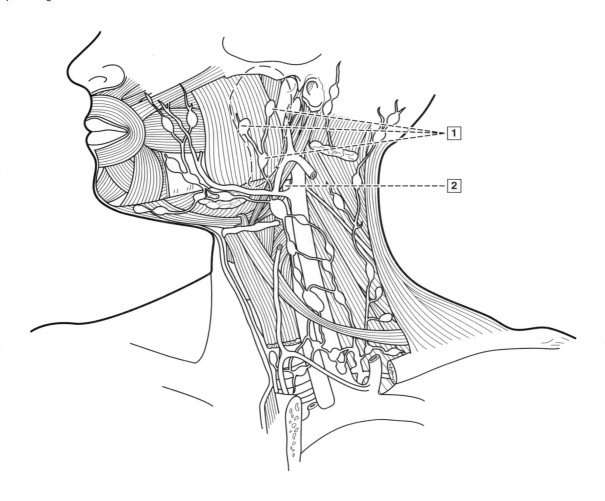

1 Deep parotid nodes

2 Retropharyngeal node

Copyright © 2008 by Saunders, an imprint of Elsevier Inc.

NOTES

Copyright © 2008 by Saunders, an imprint of Elsevier Inc.

FIGURE 9-4 | Superficial nodes of the neck (lateral view)

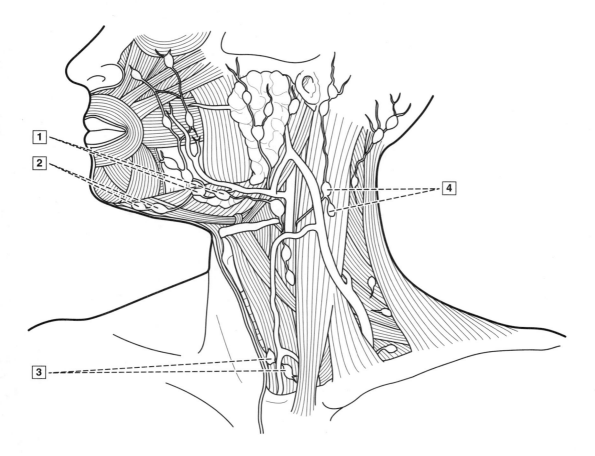

1. Submandibular nodes
2. Submental nodes
3. Anterior jugular nodes
4. External jugular nodes

Copyright © 2008 by Saunders, an imprint of Elsevier Inc.

NOTES

Copyright © 2008 by Saunders, an imprint of Elsevier Inc.

FIGURE 9-5 | Deep nodes of the neck (lateral view)

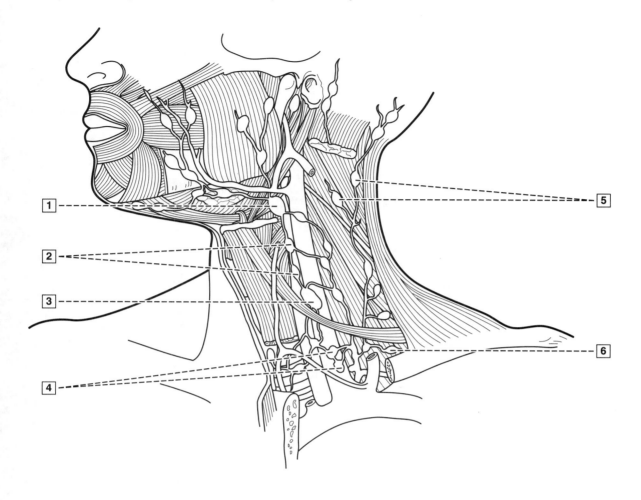

[1] Jugulodigastric node

[2] Superior deep cervical nodes

[3] Jugulo-omohyoid node

[4] Inferior deep cervical nodes

[5] Accessory nodes

[6] Supraclavicular node

NOTES

Copyright © 2008 by Saunders, an imprint of Elsevier Inc.

FIGURE 9-6 | Tonsils and associated structures (sagittal section)

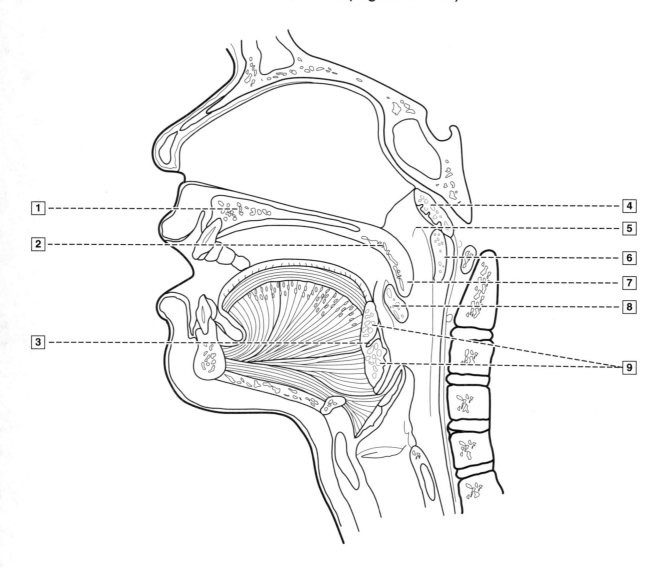

1 Hard palate	**6** Tubal tonsil
2 Soft palate	**7** Uvula
3 Foramen cecum	**8** Palatine tonsil
4 Pharyngeal tonsil	**9** Lingual tonsil
5 Opening of auditory tube	

Copyright © 2008 by Saunders, an imprint of Elsevier Inc.

NOTES

Copyright © 2008 by Saunders, an imprint of Elsevier Inc.

FIGURE 10-1 | Fasciae: face (frontal section of the head)

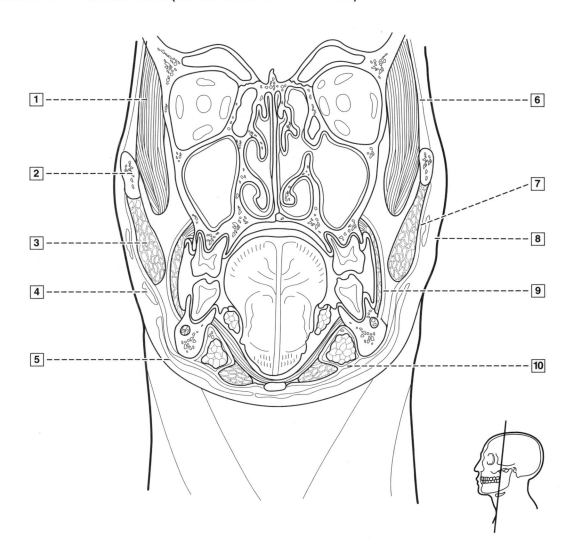

1	Temporalis muscle	**6**	Temporal fascia
2	Zygomatic bone	**7**	Masseteric-parotid fascia
3	Masseter muscle	**8**	Superficial fascia
4	Risorius muscle	**9**	Buccopharyngeal part of visceral fascia
5	Platysma muscle	**10**	Investing fascia

Copyright © 2008 by Saunders, an imprint of Elsevier Inc.

NOTES

Copyright © 2008 by Saunders, an imprint of Elsevier Inc.

FIGURE 10-2 | Fasciae: oral cavity and neck (transverse section of the oral cavity and neck)

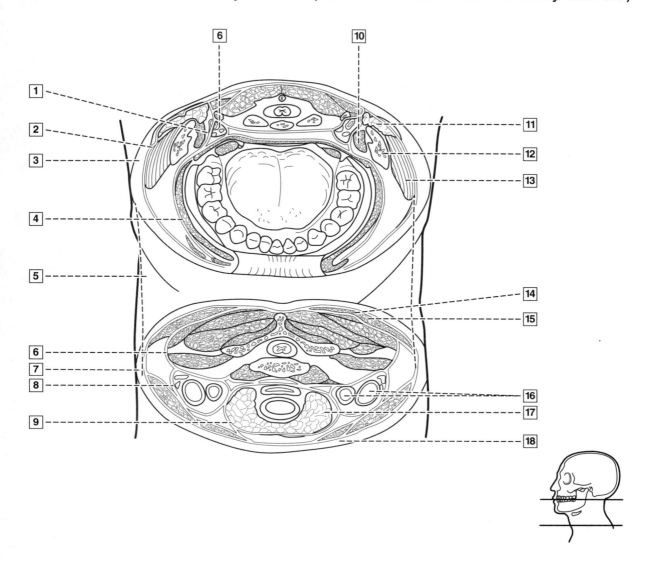

1	Pterygoid fascia	7	Investing fascia	13	Masseter muscle
2	Masseteric-parotid fascia	8	Carotid sheath	14	Trapezius muscle
3	Superficial fascia	9	Visceral fascia	15	Vertebral muscle
4	Buccopharyngeal part of visceral fascia	10	Medial pterygoid muscle	16	Internal carotid artery and internal jugular vein
5	Continuous layer	11	Parotid salivary gland	17	Thyroid gland
6	Vertebral fascia	12	Mandible	18	Platysma muscle

Copyright © 2008 by Saunders, an imprint of Elsevier Inc.

NOTES

Copyright © 2008 by Saunders, an imprint of Elsevier Inc.

FIGURE 10-3 | Fasciae: cervical fasciae (midsagittal section of the head and neck)

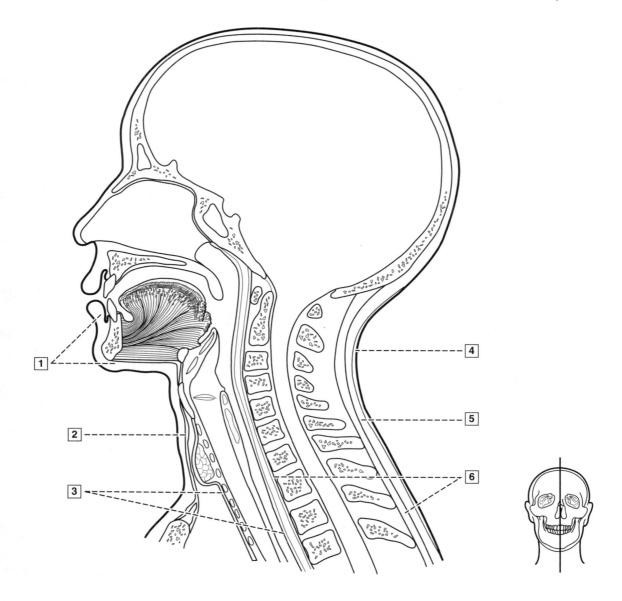

1 Superficial fascia
(with muscles of facial expression)

2 Investing fascia

3 Visceral fascia

4 Superficial fascia

5 Investing fascia

6 Vertebral fascia

Copyright © 2008 by Saunders, an imprint of Elsevier Inc.

NOTES

Copyright © 2008 by Saunders, an imprint of Elsevier Inc.

FIGURE 10-4 | Fasciae: cervical fasciae (transverse section of the neck)

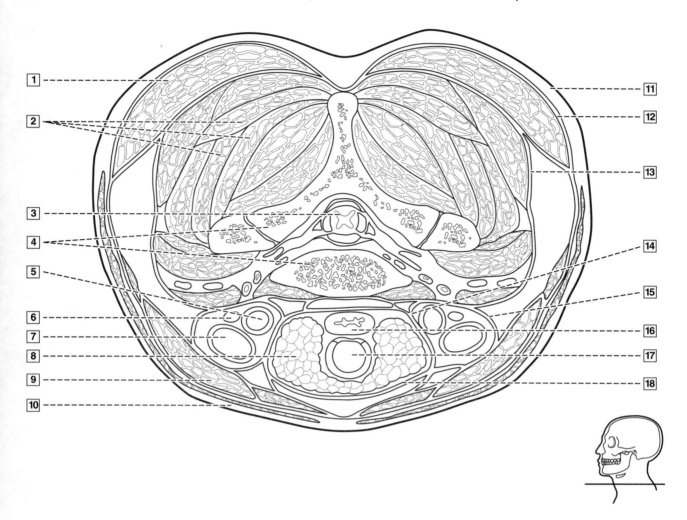

1	Trapezius muscle	7	Internal jugular vein	13	Vertebral fascia
2	Vertebral muscles	8	Thyroid gland	14	Visceral fascia
3	Spinal cord	9	Sternocleidomastoid muscle	15	Carotid sheath
4	Cervical vertebra	10	Platysma muscle	16	Esophagus
5	Common carotid artery	11	Superficial fascia	17	Trachea
6	Vagus nerve	12	Investing fascia	18	Visceral fascia

Copyright © 2008 by Saunders, an imprint of Elsevier Inc.

NOTES

Copyright © 2008 by Saunders, an imprint of Elsevier Inc.

FIGURE 10-5 | Spaces: vestibular spaces (frontal section of the head)

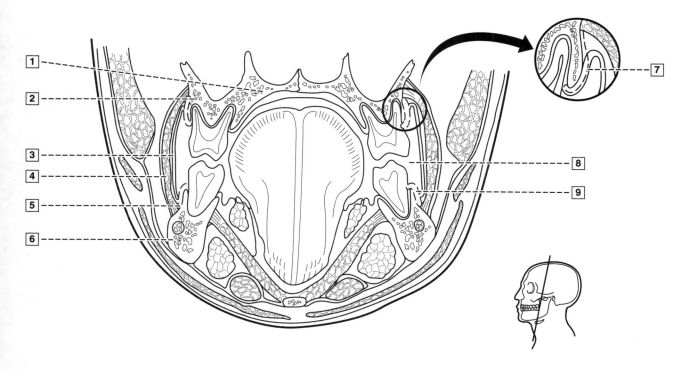

1	Palatine process of maxilla		6	Mandible
2	Alveolar process of maxilla		7	Vestibular space of maxilla
3	Oral mucosa		8	Vestibule of mouth
4	Buccinator muscle		9	Vestibular space of mandible
5	Alveolar process of mandible			

Copyright © 2008 by Saunders, an imprint of Elsevier Inc.

NOTES

Copyright © 2008 by Saunders, an imprint of Elsevier Inc.

FIGURE 10-6 | Spaces: canine and buccal spaces (frontal view of the head)

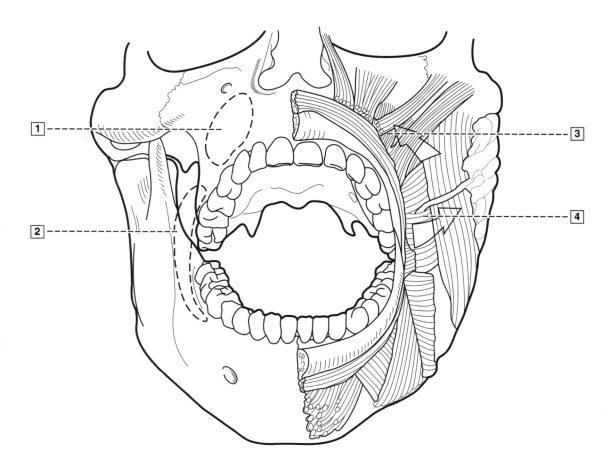

1	Canine space
2	Buccal space
3	Canine space (deep to muscles that elevate lip)
4	Buccal space (deep to masseter muscle)

Copyright © 2008 by Saunders, an imprint of Elsevier Inc.

NOTES

Copyright © 2008 by Saunders, an imprint of Elsevier Inc.

FIGURE 10-7 | Spaces: parotid space (transverse section of the head)

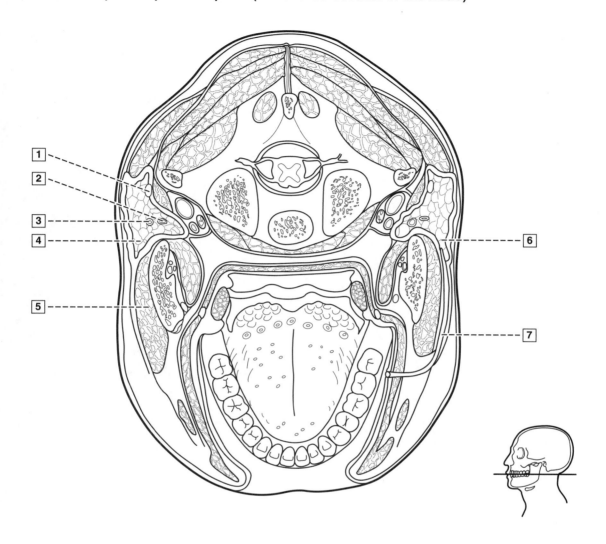

1 | Facial nerve
2 | Retromandibular vein
3 | External carotid artery
4 | Parotid salivary gland
5 | Masseter muscle
6 | Parotid space
7 | Parotid duct

Copyright © 2008 by Saunders, an imprint of Elsevier Inc.

NOTES

Copyright © 2008 by Saunders, an imprint of Elsevier Inc.

FIGURE 10-8 | Spaces: temporal and infratemporal spaces (lateral view and frontal section of the head)

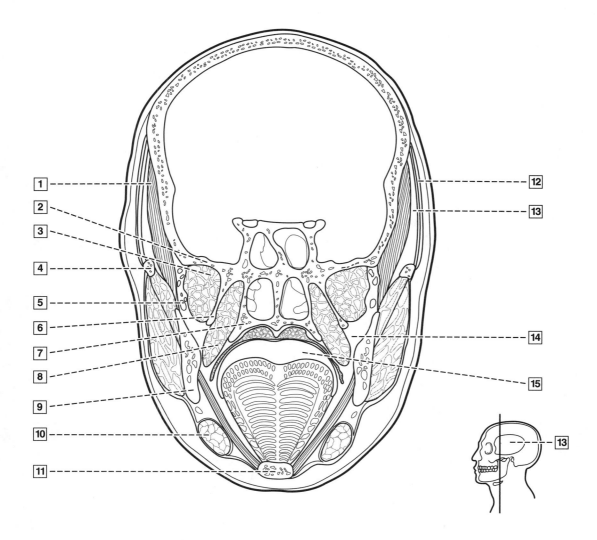

1	Temporalis muscle	9	Mandible
2	Infratemporal crest	10	Submandibular salivary gland
3	Lateral pterygoid muscle	11	Hyoid bone
4	Zygomatic bone	12	Temporal fascia
5	Maxillary artery	13	Temporal space
6	Lateral pterygoid plate	14	Infratemporal space
7	Medial pterygoid plate	15	Oral cavity
8	Medial pterygoid muscle		

Copyright © 2008 by Saunders, an imprint of Elsevier Inc.

NOTES

Copyright © 2008 by Saunders, an imprint of Elsevier Inc.

FIGURE 10-9 | Spaces: infratemporal and pterygomandibular spaces (median section of the skull)

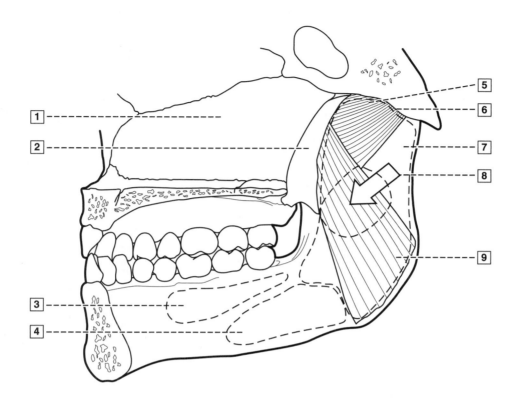

1	Vomer	**6**	Infratemporal crest
2	Medial pterygoid plate	**7**	Infratemporal space
3	Area of sublingual space	**8**	Pterygomandibular space
4	Area of submandibular space	**9**	Medial pterygoid muscle
5	Lateral pterygoid muscle		

Copyright © 2008 by Saunders, an imprint of Elsevier Inc.

NOTES

Copyright © 2008 by Saunders, an imprint of Elsevier Inc.

FIGURE 10-10 | Spaces: pterygomandibular space (transverse section of the head)

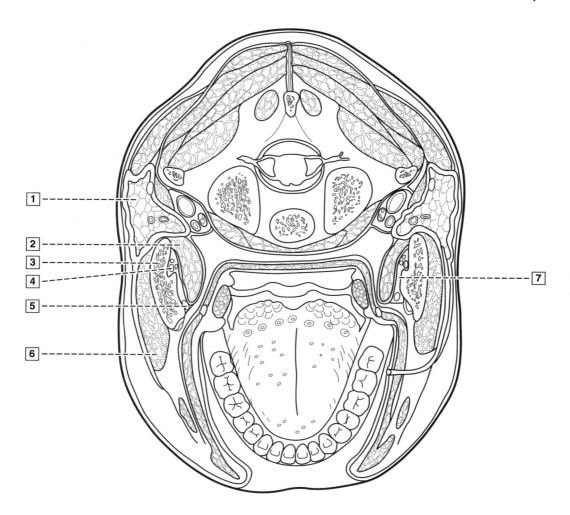

1	Parotid salivary gland
2	Medial pterygoid muscle
3	Mandible
4	Inferior alveolar nerve
5	Lingual nerve
6	Masseter muscle
7	Pterygomandibular space

NOTES

Copyright © 2008 by Saunders, an imprint of Elsevier Inc.

FIGURE 10-11 | Spaces: submasseteric space (lateral views of the face and mandible)

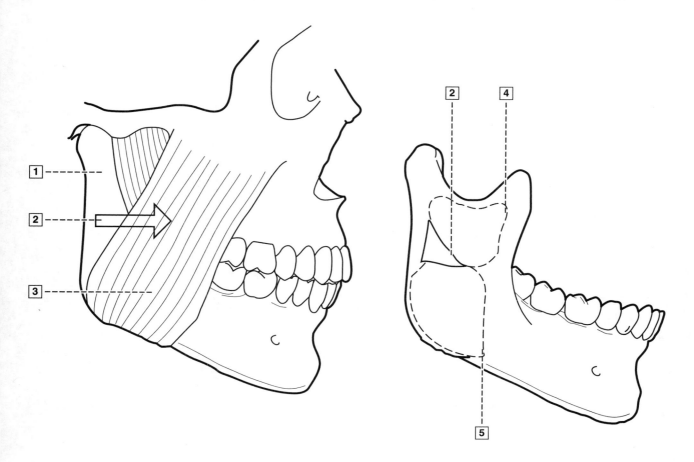

1 Ramus
2 Submasseteric space
3 Masseter muscle
4 Insertion of deep head of masseter muscle
5 Insertion of superficial head of masseter muscle

Copyright © 2008 by Saunders, an imprint of Elsevier Inc.

NOTES

Copyright © 2008 by Saunders, an imprint of Elsevier Inc.

FIGURE 10-12 │ Spaces: spaces of the mandible (frontal section of the head)

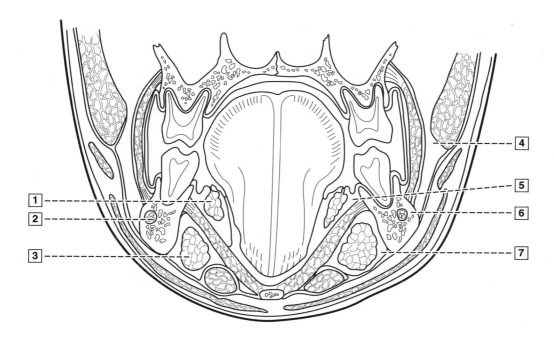

1 Sublingual salivary gland

2 Inferior alveolar nerve, artery, and vein

3 Submandibular salivary gland

4 Buccal space

5 Sublingual space

6 Space of body of mandible

7 Submandibular space

Copyright © 2008 by Saunders, an imprint of Elsevier Inc.

NOTES

Copyright © 2008 by Saunders, an imprint of Elsevier Inc.

FIGURE 10-13 | Spaces: submental and submandibular spaces (anterolateral view of the neck, with skin and platysma muscle removed)

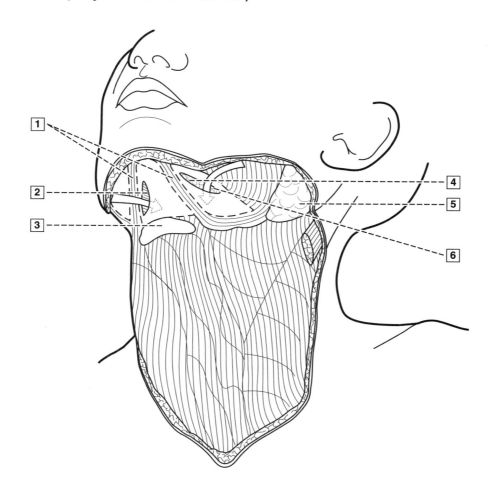

1 Anterior bellies of digastric muscle

2 Superficial cervical fascia
(cut to demonstrate entrance into submental space)

3 Hyoid bone

4 Submandibular salivary gland

5 Superficial cervical fascia
(cut to demonstrate entrance into submandibular space)

Copyright © 2008 by Saunders, an imprint of Elsevier Inc.

NOTES

Copyright © 2008 by Saunders, an imprint of Elsevier Inc.

FIGURE 10-14 | Spaces: submental and submandibular spaces (frontal section of the head and neck)

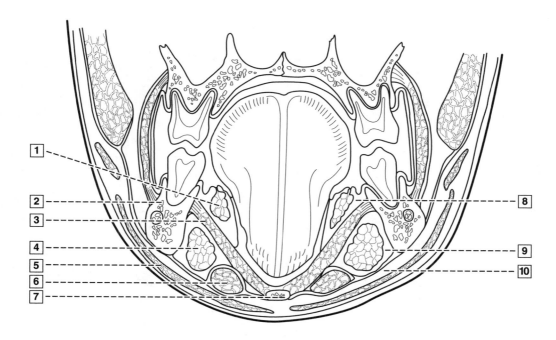

1	Sublingual salivary gland	6	Digastric muscle
2	Mandible	7	Hyoid bone
3	Mylohyoid muscle	8	Sublingual space
4	Submandibular salivary gland	9	Submandibular space
5	Platysma muscle	10	Investing fascia

Copyright © 2008 by Saunders, an imprint of Elsevier Inc.

NOTES

Copyright © 2008 by Saunders, an imprint of Elsevier Inc.

FIGURE 10-15 | Spaces: retropharyngeal and parapharyngeal spaces (transverse section of the oral cavity)

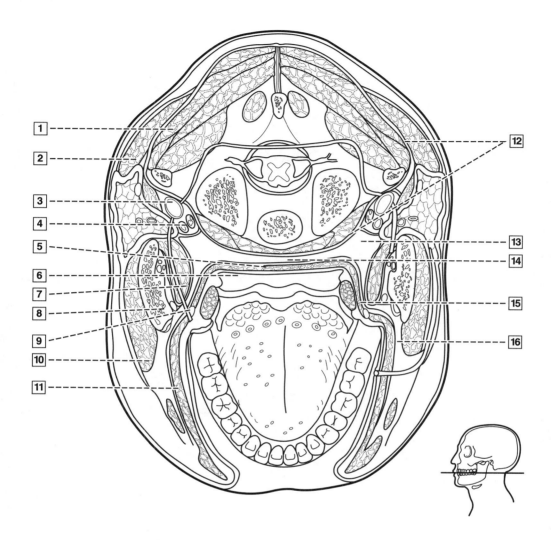

1	Vertebral muscles	9	Pterygomandibular raphe
2	Sternocleidomastoid muscle	10	Masseter muscle
3	Internal jugular vein	11	Buccinator muscle
4	Internal carotid artery	12	Vertebral fascia
5	Superior pharyngeal constrictor muscle	13	Parapharyngeal space
6	Pharynx	14	Retropharyngeal space
7	Medial pterygoid muscle	15	Buccopharyngeal fascia
8	Mandible	16	Buccal space

Copyright © 2008 by Saunders, an imprint of Elsevier Inc.

NOTES

Copyright © 2008 by Saunders, an imprint of Elsevier Inc.

FIGURE 10-16 | Spaces: retropharyngeal and previsceral spaces (midsagittal section of the head and neck)

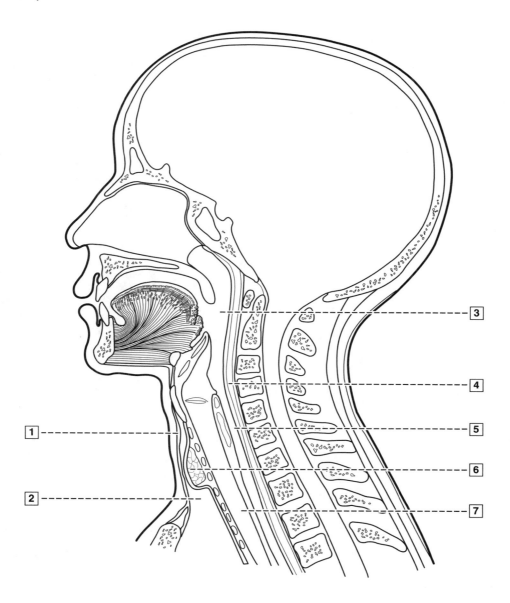

1 Investing fascia

2 Previsceral space

3 Pharynx

4 Retropharyngeal space

5 Esophagus

6 Thyroid gland

7 Trachea

Copyright © 2008 by Saunders, an imprint of Elsevier Inc.

NOTES

Copyright © 2008 by Saunders, an imprint of Elsevier Inc.

FIGURE 10-17 | Spaces: retropharyngeal and previsceral spaces (transverse section of the neck)

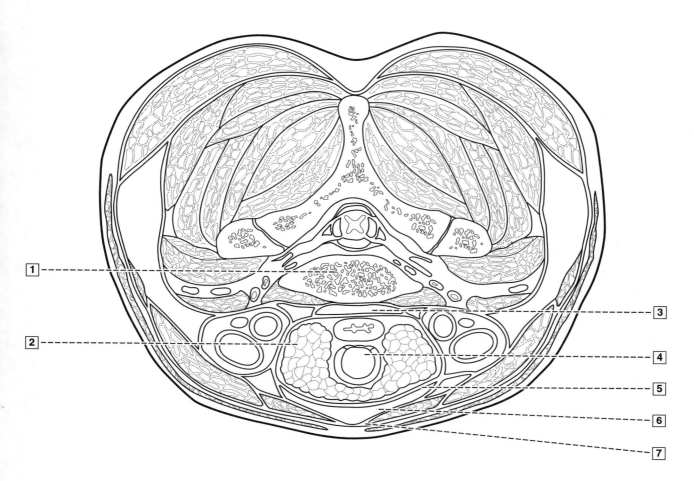

1 Cervical vertebrae
2 Thyroid gland
3 Retropharyngeal space
4 Trachea
5 Visceral fascia
6 Previsceral space
7 Investing fascia

Copyright © 2008 by Saunders, an imprint of Elsevier Inc.

NOTES

Copyright © 2008 by Saunders, an imprint of Elsevier Inc.